BABY
designed
by God

DR
AMANDA HESS

DR
JEREMY HESS

Boise, Idaho

RM RUSSELL
MEDIA

Published in Boise, Idaho by Russell Media
www.russell-media.com

This book may be purchased in bulk for educational, business, ministry, or promotional use.

For information please email: info@russell-media.com.

ISBN (print): 978-1-937498-42-9
ISBN (e-book): 978-1-937498-43-6

Printed in the United States of America

For all the women who pray and long
for the miracle of birth.
For them to achieve the birth of their dreams.

To raising up children in the way they should go.
Not only our children, Alyssa and Gabriel,
but for all of God's children to have the opportunity
to live out their God-given birth-right to be healthy
and whole, just the way they were created!

We are forever grateful to God for bestowing on us
the knowledge of the innate principle of health, life
and healing from the inside-out.

– Drs. Amanda and Jeremy Hess

Endorsements and Praise

"I personally know of no other individuals who understand the idea that the human body is a temple of the Holy Spirit better than Drs. Amanda and Jeremy Hess. Their passion and knowledge is revolutionizing audiences across the nation in the areas of healthy living and raising drug free children. The sooner that families can be exposed to these truths the better...this book is a Godsend."

Gregg Kennard
NSPIRE Outreach

"Drs.Jeremy and Amanda Hess' book *Baby Designed By God* explains how expecting parents can use God-given innate wisdom to confidently nurture their children toward better health. This book is extremely informative and insightful while offering practical steps for parents to take. I recommend it!"

Dr. Beau Adams
Lead Pastor, Community Bible Church

"Dr.'s Jeremy and Amanda Hess, two of the most successful chiropractors of this generation, have written a GEM! Through the pages of *Baby Designed By God*, you will be enlightened to the intricacies and magnificence of human life and what it takes to truly get healthy and stay healthy!"

Dr. Pete Sulack
Author of Fellowshipping with God's Voice
Matthew 10 Ministries - matthew10.com

"Drs. Jeremy and Amanda Hess' book, Baby Designed By God, shows parents how to use wisdom and health principles in teaching and raising up their children towards a life of health that God desires for them to have. This book is a must read for any parent who is uncertain about the 'status quo' of our healthcare culture and wants their child to live a drug free, vibrant and healthy life."

Michael Turner
Sr. Pastor of Turning Point Church
Author of *Watch Me Daddy*

"The *Design by God* series is a necessity in every home. The natural health principles shared are right on and if practiced by families on a regular basis would shift the health of our country for generations to come. Drs. Jeremy & Amanda Hess hit it out of the park...it's MUST read."

Dr. Michael Viscarelli,
ADIO Chiropractic
Golden, Colorado

"Every time I'm with Drs. Amanda and Jeremy Hess, I always feel a lot better afterward! That's because they are passionate about helping people experience optimum health. But this book may disturb you. In it, they challenge 'conventional wisdom' often espoused by doctors, nurses, and hospitals. You owe it to yourself and your children to read this book!"

Dr. Richard Blackaby
Author of *The Inspired Leader, Experiencing God at Home* and *The Seasons of God*

"A straightforward manuel that includes simple steps for birthing and raising your child in an over medicated society."

Meri Warbrick, RDH,ND

"*Baby Designed by God* is a must read for current and future parents. Filled with well researched information yet still a joy to read, Drs. Jeremy and Amanda Hess have put together a book that can help everyone become informed about their choices for their bodies and their babies. We cannot wait to read the next one in the series!"

Dr. Erik Brower and Mrs. Dana Brower, MAT

"Empowering, eye-opening, and honest! *Baby Designed by God* is unlike any other pregnancy book on the market today!"

Charity Haulk
Natural Child Birth Educator

table of contents

1.
Expecting a Miracle

Oh yes, you shaped me first inside, then out; you formed me in my mother's womb. I thank you, High God— you're breathtaking! Body and soul, I am marvelously made! I worship in adoration—what a creation! You know me inside and out, you know every bone in my body; You know exactly how I was made, bit by bit, how I was sculpted from nothing into something. Like an open book, you watched me grow from conception to birth; all the stages of my life were spread out before you, the days of my life all prepared before I'd even lived one day. Psalm 139:13-16 (The Message *translation)*

A Miracle in the Making

"So, do you think it's a boy or a girl?" Isn't that always the question posed to a new mom or dad, whether to take stock in pinks or blues, dolls or trucks and trains! But the answer is always the same: "Just as long as it's healthy, that's all we're hoping and praying for." Every parent carries the innate desire

11

to have children with ten fingers and ten toes, eyes that see and a smile and giggle that glows. That's the expected miracle we all yearn for as soon-to-be moms and dads, from the moment we find out we are expecting.

By definition, a miracle is "a surprising and welcome event that is not explicable by natural or scientific laws and is considered to be divine." We love this definition because it describes the conception, development and birth of a baby perfectly—a divine event, simply a miracle. As you read this, consider yourself one of those miracles. When your mother and father were together moments before conception, millions of sperm from dad were rushing to meet up with your mother's egg and one of those sperm amongst the millions was you. You're the one that made it and you are living proof of the magnificence of God's creation and the perfection of the process. The infinite number of developmental steps that have to take place from conception to birth is truly unfathomable and remarkable!

Most pregnant moms take for granted the all-encompassing miracle that takes place in the womb. Already on day 6, the embryo begins implantation in the uterus. By the third week, the heart begins to beat with the child's own blood, often a different type than the mother's. The child's brain stem, spinal column and nervous system are forming and the liver, kidneys and intestines begin to take shape. By the end of week four, the child is ten thousand times larger than the fertilized egg. In the fifth week, its eyes, legs and hands begin to develop.

At only six weeks old and in many cases about the time mom realizes she's pregnant, brain waves are detectable, mouth and lips are present and fingers are forming. In week 7, distinct eyelids, toes and a nose develop. The baby is now kicking and swimming. At week 8, every organ is in place, bones begin to replace cartilage and fingerprints begin to form and the baby can begin to hear. In weeks 9, 10 and 11, teeth begin to form, fingernails develop. The baby can turn his head, frown and hiccup. He or she can also "breathe" amniotic fluid and urinate and can grasp objects placed in its hand; all his organ systems are functioning. The baby has a skeletal structure, nerves and circulation.

By week 12, the baby has all of the parts necessary to experience pain, including nerves, spinal cord and thalamus. Vocal cords are complete and the baby can suck its thumb. At the age of 14 weeks, the heart pumps several quarts of blood through the body every day and the baby has adult taste buds by 15 weeks old. When the baby reaches four months, bone marrow is now beginning to form and the heart is pumping 25 quarts of blood per day. By the end of month 4, the baby will be eight to ten inches in length and will weigh up to half a pound; about that time, he or she can have dream (REM) sleep.

At 20 weeks, the baby recognizes its mother's voice. By months 5 and 6, the baby practices breathing by inhaling amniotic fluid into its developing lungs and the baby will grasp at the umbilical cord when it feels it. Most mothers feel an increase in movement, kicking and hiccups from the baby. Oil and sweat glands are now functioning. The baby is now twelve inches long or more and weighs up to one and a half pounds. During months 7 through 9, the baby opens and closes his or her eyes and is using four of the five senses (vision, hearing, taste and touch). He or she knows the difference between waking and sleeping and can relate to the moods of his mother. The baby's skin begins to thicken and a layer of fat is produced and stored beneath the skin. Antibodies are built up and the baby's heart begins to pump 300 gallons of blood per day. Approximately one week before birth, the baby stops growing and "drops" into the pelvic cavity.[1] Amazingly, this entire process transpires without anyone orchestrating it or having to plan it.

Another natural process that requires no orchestrating or planning that God gave each woman is her "motherly intuition." In our opinion, a mother's intuition is the internal sixth sense that we believe God gives every woman to help her mentally, physically and emotionally handle every challenge and decision that comes with bearing and rearing children. It's sometimes the "wee small voice" that tells mom something feels right or wrong. It's also the crucial decision to do one thing, even though others are saying to do another. Over the years, our health culture has started to question a mother's intuition, or to urge a mother to act in direct opposition to what she feels and knows is right.

We encountered this kind of current cultural mentality at our first baby shower, when some well-meaning ladies from the church gave us a book on how to put our baby on an infant training schedule of feeding and sleeping. The "baby" was not in control of us; we would stay in control of the baby. As we read the book, some of the recommendations just didn't sit right with us. Maybe you've been in the same situation where you were instructed to just let the baby cry it out while you sheepishly tried to ignore it, or your intuition told you that your baby is hungry, but your best friend (who follows the "schedule your

---

[1] http://www.nrlc.org/abortion/facts/fetaldevelopment.html

baby doctrine") made you feel the baby was taking advantage of you. Always follow your God-given maternal intuition. Just because the herd is doing something does not mean that you have to follow suit. You are your own person and God chose you to be your baby's best advocate.

It's commonly understood that all babies, whether humans or animals, are helpless to do anything for themselves. They completely depend on mom for nourishment through breastfeeding or bottle-feeding and have the need of intimate handling and touch from their caregivers. As a fetus, the baby just spent 9 months in its mom's womb, which is a wonderful, warm, dark, quiet and fluid environment. Wouldn't everyone want to spend at least a couple of days vacationing in warm water, where it is dark and quiet with no disturbances—it seems like paradise! Then, all of a sudden, the baby comes out into a cold, brightly lit, dry environment. It only makes sense that the baby wants to be held by mom, feel her warmth and touch, suckle her breast for food and be rocked back and forth just as he or she was in the womb. The idea of letting the baby cry it out or not feeding the baby because it was hungry before the pre-set time interval just seemed absurd to us. Thankfully, we felt vindicated with our parental intuition after reading the book *Boundaries* by Dr. Henry Cloud and Dr. John Townsend.

Designed by God?

We vividly remember the birth of our children. We witnessed their first breath outside the womb, the first time they looked us in the eyes and we connected and the sight of the blood still passing through the cord from mom's body to theirs. They had the innate instinct to nurse, to be held and to bond with us. How could our babies' bodies know how to breathe on their own, to produce liver enzymes, or to digest mother's milk? How does a baby's immune system know to start protecting itself from the second it enters the world? Who told the baby's heart, kidneys and pituitary gland to function?

We believe God designed our bodies wonderfully and magnificently in His image, giving them everything they need. If that isn't the case, then why even be born? God provides our bodies with an internal, innate intelligence so they know exactly what to do, when to do it, how to function and how to meet all of our needs. This God-given capability of our bodies to control and coordinate all bodily functions begins at the time of conception and leaves us at the time of death. It works around the clock, even while we are asleep: making our heart beat, causing a fever in our body when we need to fight an infection, keeping digestion moving, activating the sweat glands when we get hot or causing us to shiver when we get cold, creating enzymes and acids, balancing the body chemistry and on and on. Because our babies grow and change so much from conception to the toddler years, this internal intelligence as the residing factor is very evident and gives God the credit and glory. Even to the non-believer, this divine design just makes sense.

Then, something happens. Usually not all at once, but slowly and gradually, we are broken down by our current health culture, spurred on by the media and societal trends. The idea creeps into our minds that we are born into this world incomplete, that God didn't give us everything we needed and that we require artificial substances and procedures from outside of our bodies to be made whole once again. For some of us and our babies, it happens fairly soon after delivery, as hospitals and doctors question our body's ability to care for itself, to heal and grow, or even to provide us with the basic necessities of life.

This faulty mentality lies at the core of why we wrote this book and it's the essence of the unraveling of our health culture, which treats and looks at the body from the outside in. It says that our bodies were designed by God to fail and not to thrive, that we weren't wonderfully and magnificently made, that we are guilty as charged when it comes to being diseased—including the miracle of pregnancy.

For many women, this culture says that health comes from a pill bottle, potion, or lotion and it teaches them that God didn't provide completely for our babies' immune system, so they are lacking "protection." This concept that a newborn child is immediately susceptible to death and disease is most apparent after delivery, as newborns are injected with all kinds of foreign substances, such as vaccinations, in the false belief system that the baby will die or suffer permanent damage without them. The actions taken on our babies and children speak volumes about our "healthcare" system and how our current culture and society views health, healing, sickness and disease. Our mission is to resurrect and bring about change to a generation, to teach the fundamentals of health and healing from the inside out, to once again bring to the forefront that not only our babies, but all of us are designed by God, in His image and in His perfection.

A Healthy Perspective

Evidence of humanity's will to be well dates back to over 5000 years ago with Imhotep, a man who was considered the "Great Physician of Egypt." He took records and wrote prescriptions, or "healing formulas," on papyrus. He also transcribed the basic rudiments of health: *a sensible diet, a steady mind, cleanliness, mental activity and devotion to universal law* (or, shall we say in our understanding now, a devotion to God as the designer and creator). Now, Imhotep's understanding was quite unique and modern, so ahead of his time that we still have not caught up with it in the present day.[2] Most of us are taught quite differently. Culturally, it's normal to be sick and expect disease. We are taught from an early age to cover up symptoms and self-medicate. It starts with whatever we already have in the medicine cabinet, then the pharmacy if we need something more potent and then the doctor to get a prescription. This approach to the suppression of our symptoms is all around us.

As we watch TV, browse the Internet, or read magazines, pharmaceutical ads are everywhere. Studies report that close to every third ad on TV promotes a pharmaceutical drug. *Medical News Today* research found that Americans watch up to 16 hours of TV ads about prescription drugs per week. They also discovered that New Zealand and the United States are the only developed countries that allow prescription drugs to be advertised directly to the consumer via television. New Zealand is considering stopping it.[3] When we were children in the 1980s, our parents always had a subscription to *Prevention* magazine

---

[2] *The Chiropractic Story*, by Marcus Bach
[3] http://www.medicalnewstoday.com/articles/61985.php

and it published good information, articles and editorials about relevant health topics.

Now, flipping through an issue of *Prevention* or *Reader's Digest* reveals advertisements peddling and promoting the latest fad drugs to Americans at an alarming rate. Unfortunately, it gets worse. Now, many medical doctors and medical journals like the *British Medical Journal* are reporting on "disease mongering." Pharmaceutical companies actually create diseases and then magically produce the antidotes for the same diseases they've just invented. With these "new" diseases, pharmaceutical companies increase their profits by convincing essentially well people that they are sick, or slightly sick people that they are very ill.

Most families don't recognize the seeds of pharmaceutical propaganda; however, in our family, we try to combat this disturbing topic by educating our children. About a year ago, when our daughter Alyssa was in kindergarten, she came to us one day and told us that she had to bring one of her stuffed bears to class. This seemed out of the ordinary because the teacher didn't normally allow toys in class, so we asked why. Alyssa then told us that the class was to give their stuffed animals "flu shots." To say we were appalled and shocked would be an understatement! Alyssa, in her 5-year-old mindset, just laughed and told us, "Mommy, Daddy, it's just pretend. I know that we don't get shots, but everybody else in the class says they do. So let me take my bear and I'll just do what the teacher says, because that's what I'm supposed to do."

This exposure only continues when our kids come home from school and watch TV. Simply put, wherever they go, our children are bombarded daily with fast food, processed junk food ads and pharmaceutical drug ads on TV, the Internet and even just riding around town.

Even the schools have a sick care mentality and don't want to be bothered with symptoms. The school nurse's office is no longer the place to just get your temperature taken, lay down if you're not feeling well and get a Band-Aid for a scrape. In most cases, the nurse is similar to a pharmacy technician distributing out medicines that kids take on a daily basis for allergies, asthma, reflux, attention deficit hyperactivity disorder and so on. The nurse labels your child sick if he or she has a fever, vomits, or is coughing too much.

We remember recently having to pick up our daughter one day at noon due to a temperature; however, after receiving her chiropractic adjustment and taking a three hour nap, she woke up refreshed and ready to play. She definitely could have returned to school the following morning and been fine; however, we had to wait until after twelve o'clock the next day before the school would accept our child, as they had a 24-hour "waiting period" on fevers. By mid-day, what's the point of sending her at all? She basically missed a day of education even though she was perfectly fine.

Many people get anxious about fevers only because they have been wrongly informed that a fever is always a bad thing and requires immediate intervention and medication. However, God created fevers for a reason. Essentially, fevers are the body's normal physiological mechanism to kill foreign substances, such as bacteria or viruses, by increasing the body's internal temperature. By artificially lowering a fever with a pill, you are interfering with the body's natural ability to heal itself, which may cause the fever and symptoms to linger.

The physiological responses surrounding vomiting and diarrhea also have garnered unnecessary criticism. On rare occasions, we have had to pick up our children at school after one of them has vomited because "that's the rule"—if you vomit, you're out. We remember one particular late morning, where one of us had to leave work to rescue our supposedly contagious, sickly child, only to pick her up, get in the car and hear the words, "Mommy, can we go to Starbucks now? I feel great!" Just recently we visited Disney World and while waiting to ride Aladdin's carpet ride, our son said he had to go "poo-poo." I asked him to wait as we were at the front of the line and he said "okay". So we got on the ride and as soon as we got off, he asked again but this time with a grimace on his face. My intuition told me that this is not good. So I picked him up, ran to the nearest bathroom and watched him have diarrhea for the next 10 minutes while crying out in pain as his stomach and colon were cramping. My first thought as this was happening was that vacation was over and we would be heading immediately back to the hotel. But I knew that the diarrhea was just the body's natural way to rid itself of toxins.

So after the 10 minutes of sitting on the toilet and asking my three year old if he thought that was all of it, he stood up off the toilet, wanted to drink a lot of water (probably from some dehydration) and asked to go see the pirates. I gave him a high-five and he asked for Daddy to carry him on his shoulders to see the pirates. The common belief system is if you vomit, cough or have diarrhea, you must be sick. Our belief system is that God created the body to have these symptoms when necessary to remove toxins and disagreeable substances from the body.

Neither vomiting nor fever are signs of disease, but often they indicate that the body is doing exactly what it is supposed to do. We're not saying all fevers, diarrhea and/or vomiting fall into this category, but the vast majority do. Yes, there are real cases of medical emergencies that need proper care; however, most of fevers, colds and stomach concerns don't require medical or over-the-counter solutions. They require rest, a well-functioning nervous system and proper nutrition and hydration.

In order to counter the ideas of modern, mainstream belief systems, we teach our children the principles of right and wrong and the importance of being respectful and we discipline when necessary; we try our best to mold them into the individuals that God wants them to be. Likewise, to counter the ideas of the modern, mainstream medical culture, we also teach our children about health, living naturally and health and healing from the inside out. We teach them about good versus bad foods—or, as we call the good foods in our home, foods from the earth or God, versus the bad foods, foods from man or processed foods. We try to explain the difference between organic, healthy good choices and processed, fast food and bad choices. We fight an uphill, daily battle to train our children in the way they should go.

In the United States of America, when most of our babies leave the womb, they are in the middle of the best "health care" in the world, right? Or are they? Research from May 2013 states that the United States has the highest first-day infant mortality rate of any of the 68 other countries in the industrialized world.

This statistic means that more babies are dying here than in any of those other 68 countries on day one of the baby's life. Not only that, but the United States' rate of first-day infant death is 50 percent higher than all the other industrialized countries combined.

We keep referring to the terms inside-out and outside-in and in essence, this terminology differentiates "health care" versus "sick care." Our bodies naturally heal from the inside out. God gave them everything they need on the inside, wonderfully and magnificently making them in His image? Anything that we might put in them, like organic, whole foods, herbs, or natural substances are there to help the body function normally and allow it to heal from the inside out. Outside-in treatment attempts to fix the body with artificial, man-made substances, things like ointments, potions, toxic treatments and pharmaceutical drugs. The outside-in approach is always trying to determine how to control the body's function from a drug, pill, or procedure. It says, "Man's educated system knows more than the internal wisdom that God put inside of you when you were conceived." With these two opposing practices on how to view the body and its function, we end up with two very different protocols of how to care for the human body and its possible ailments.

What we now know as our health care system is really a system of "sick care." Sick care waits for symptoms to show up before anything is done, because in the sick care model, if you don't have any symptoms, then that means you're healthy. Sick care also suggests that if you do have symptoms, it means you're sick and need treatment.

Many times, the sick care model is based on **F.E.A.R.**, which means, **F**alse **E**vidence **A**ppearing **R**eal. Sick care teaches us not to trust the body's intelligent mechanisms that God put within us. It also teaches us to expect the worst and, though it may appear well-meaning, it destroys our faith that God made our bodies and can heal them, which makes us feel completely helpless.

Let's look at this sick care understanding of symptoms more closely. Imagine you have two co-workers, Susan and Betty, who are both in their 40s. First, let's look at Susan. You see her at work often. She looks good, she's in pretty good shape, has an upbeat attitude and seems healthy. If I asked you if she was healthy, you probably would say she is. Susan probably would say she's healthy too. But what Susan and you both don't know is that she is in the early stages of breast cancer. She doesn't know this because she shows no signs of cancer, not even on a mammogram. Knowing this, would you say she is healthy or sick? Obviously, now you would say she is sick and not well. Betty, on the other hand, misses work for two days and you hear that she was at home with diarrhea, vomiting and nausea. You immediately would say she is sick. Now, what you didn't know was that Betty ate some food at a local restaurant, where she got food poisoning. Her body is reacting normally by ridding her body of toxins through the vomiting and diarrhea. So, is she sick, or is her body functioning normally by eliminating all the toxins from her system? Who is sick and who is healthy, Susan or Betty?

The point of this story is to show us that having symptoms isn't always a bad thing and in many cases, the symptoms mean

Prescription Drugs

More than 25% of Kids & Teens in the U.S. take Prescription Drugs on a Regular Basis

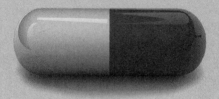

The average child in the U.S. under the age of 18 filled an average of 4.1 prescriptions in 2011. Clearly more drugs have not led to better health. Actually, the opposite has happened. (1 out of 4 kids are on a pharmaceutical regularly!)

your body is healing itself from the inside out. Remember, there is always a price to pay for suppressing symptoms with drugs. You may not see it immediately, but eventually, what you sow is what you reap and every time we put an artificial drug into our bodies or our baby's body, it damages cells and tissue. All drugs, whether pushed or prescribed, have side effects.

Similarly, if your baby is coughing or sneezing, should we "suppress" it with over-the-counter suppressants and allow the "bacteria and toxins" to stay in your baby, or allow the baby to cough and sneeze out what it needs to so it can function normally? When your baby starts to teethe, it's very common for him or her to get a fever, runny nose and excessive mucus. In our current "sick care" model, most pediatricians and "your new baby" books would tell you to use some type of drug, usually an over the counter acetaminophen (such as Tylenol) to help lower the fever and bring down his body temperature. [4]

As we mentioned earlier, the purpose of a fever is to raise the body's temperature enough to kill off certain bacteria and viruses sensitive to temperature changes. Think about it: your baby is teething and the incoming teeth cut the gums, so now there is the chance of an infection. However, because God created your baby with everything it needed when it was born, its internal mechanisms know to raise the body's temperature to a point to where it will kill off bacteria and viruses in the open wound from the incoming tooth, thus allowing your child to stay well. That's true "healthcare", allowing the body to react naturally and normally like God designed it to.

---

[4] http://drugs.about.com/lw/Health-Medicine/Drugs-and-treatments/In-the-Drugstore-OTC-Medications-to-Reduce-Fever-What-You-Need-to-Know-for-You-and-Your-Child.htm

True healthcare acknowledges that your baby is a miracle and that the body has an internal, innate intelligence given to it by God. It can regulate, control all body functions and repair and heal itself when necessary without the use of drugs or surgery. We trust and believe that God constructed us perfectly in His image. And where does it all begin? Inside every baby, because every baby is designed by God!

Alyssa's Birth Story
by Amanda Hess

In the summer of 2006 after returning from vacation, I found out I was pregnant with our first child. Immediately I knew that Jeremy and I would need to find a midwife as our primary care provider, since we had already planned on having a homebirth delivery. We also had to find an obstetrician that would accept me for prenatal care in case of the need for emergency transport to a hospital during the delivery. As both of us are chiropractors and already had the knowledge of natural childbirth versus the allopathic, medicated birth, we were informed and in agreement that having a homebirth was the direction we wanted for ourselves and our baby.

At the beginning of the pregnancy, my midwives scheduled appointments once a month to monitor my progression. I was weighed, measured, blood pressure checked, given a blood panel, administered urine samples and the baby's heartbeat was monitored by a fetoscope. Toward the end of the pregnancy, I began to see my midwives every other week and then weekly. My midwives offered all the same testing and procedures that one would receive with a licensed OBGYN; however, I remember receiving a packet of information to take home and read regarding all the various testing offered while pregnant, in the case that I felt I wanted to decline certain procedures.

I thankfully was accepted as a patient by a local obstetrician. He knew that my ultimate goal was to have a homebirth and he would only be needed in the 12 percent chance of complications during the delivery resulting in transportation to the nearest hospital for intervention. I saw him once at the beginning of the pregnancy to establish myself as a patient and during the course of my prenatal care with my midwives, there were no indications that I would be considered high risk. He knew my midwives and the care that they would give me during the pregnancy, so he asked if I wanted to schedule the second trimester check-up with him for the ultrasound (which we declined); otherwise, he would see me at 35 weeks for a final check-up before delivery.

The pregnancy went well. I received regular specific scientific chiropractic adjustments from my husband, which kept my spine and pelvis in proper alignment. I had no pain, though I suffered nausea on a few occasions. Overall, I felt normal and great, excluding the increasing size of my belly and some fatigue. My blood panel was normal; my blood pressure was normal; I was measuring normally throughout the duration of the pregnancy. The heartbeat of the baby was normal and I gained a total of 42 pounds. My urine continued to be the only concern, with leukocytes always appearing on the test strip. I continued to be asymptomatic, however and learned that there are various reasons leukocytes could appear in the urine and that it doesn't always need to cause alarm, especially during pregnancy. At the end of my pregnancy, I also tested positive for GBS (Group B streptococcus). The medical model regarding this testing would be to intervene immediately and administer intravenous antibiotics during delivery, even though testing positive for GBS does not necessarily mean that your baby will be affected. Contrary to the medical protocol of immediate intervention, my midwives informed me that there were natural homeopathic remedies that could be taken on my part to decrease the chance of GBS affecting my baby. With the desire to live as naturally as possible and the understanding that God is our provider, this was the perfect solution for me.

At 35 weeks, I returned to my obstetrician, who did the same testing of my urine, blood pressure, weight, measurements and he listened to the baby's heartbeat. He then wished me well and said with a smile, "Have a great homebirth. I probably won't see you again, but you have my number just in case."

On Tuesday, April 10, 2007, I woke up to go to the bathroom at 2:30 am. With my first step out of bed, I felt a gush of fluid in my underwear and down my legs. Then I sat on the toilet and saw a large red clump in the toilet, which was the mucous plug. I thought for sure that my water had broke, so I called my midwife, Claudia. She asked me if I felt any contractions. Since I did not, Claudia told me to go back to sleep and that she would come to the house around noon to examine me.

When I woke up later that Tuesday morning, my husband and I decided to go for a walk around the neighborhood lake in hopes that labor would begin. About every 15 minutes, I felt a twinge in my abdomen. I had to lean over or squat to help relieve the pain. After we finished our walk, Claudia arrived to check on me. Upon examining me, Claudia believed that the water was still intact and had not broken. My husband and myself already thought labor had begun and had gone ahead and cancelled all practice member appointments in our office for Tuesday and Wednesday. To our dismay, Claudia said that since the water had not broken, it could be days or even weeks for the delivery to occur. Claudia left the house and said to call her around dinnertime for an update. This was not good news to us. We had already cancelled all our practice members and for me to not be in labor was just unacceptable to us, so later that afternoon we decided to go for another walk around the lake in the hopes of speeding up this process. The contractions started to get stronger and we had to turn around and head back home. I was on our neighborhood street literally on my hands and knees in pain, so Jeremy suggested, "I think it's about time we head back inside."

We ate lasagna for dinner and started to watch The Simpsons on television. I called Claudia and told her that the contractions were about ten minutes apart. Claudia said I should probably just watch some TV and go to bed. She wanted to make sure that I got plenty of rest. As we relaxed at the house, the contractions started to get closer together and more uncomfortable. We got ready for bed and the contractions got even stronger. I kept thinking to myself that Claudia had told me to go to bed. However, Jeremy looked at me and said that my face and body looked uncomfortable and he was timing the contractions at about five minutes apart. I wanted to wait a little while longer before calling Claudia, but he wanted me to call her immediately. I gave in to my husband's request and called Claudia. She said that she was expecting my call and that she and her apprentice would be at the house soon.

Claudia and her apprentice, Nicole, arrived just after midnight on Wednesday, April 11. I was on the bed lying on my side to try to ease the pain. Claudia and Nicole examined me and started to prepare for the delivery. They set up the inflatable pool with warm water for the water birth while I went to the bathroom, where I was on my hands and knees, trying again to ease the pain. Finally, the pool was ready and everyone helped me get situated in the water. To my amazement, the water felt warm and relaxing. I started to smile instead of grimace in pain. The warm water eased up the contractions and I had a few minutes of what I call birthing paradise. This "paradise," however, was short lived. Within a few minutes, the contractions started again.

Nicole monitored me during and between the contractions, while Claudia decided to get some sleep in the guest bedroom. Between contractions, I was so embarrassed because I was burping constantly. The grossest thing about my burping was that it tasted like lasagna. I thought for sure I was going to vomit. Jeremy, however, kept encouraging me, telling me I could do this, to just keep going. He has always been and still is such a motivator. He also stood by my side the entire time making sure I continued to drink some water or juice between every contraction to keep me hydrated.

After what seemed like forever, Nicole decided to wake up Claudia and they said that it was time to push. I could feel the baby's head in the vaginal canal and after many pushes later, I thought that the head felt like it hadn't moved any further. Claudia must have been thinking the same thing, because she told me that I was too comfortable in the water and wasn't progressing enough. She encouraged me to get out of the water and onto the birthing stool. I agreed and got on the birthing stool, with Jeremy standing behind me helping to hold me up. Immediately out of my warm water, the contractions and the pushing went to the highest level of pain and intensity. I thought to myself, "This is it. I can do this. We're about to have our baby." Jeremy kept telling me to keep going, that I had just a little bit more to go. To this day, his encouraging words and him holding me up, holding my hands and doing whatever was necessary helped me to never have a moment of doubt during the delivery process.

After many more pushes, Claudia said that the water sack had still not broken and asked me if she could break it to help speed things along. I agreed and with a little pinch, the water broke. From there, everything seemed to happen so fast. I felt the baby's head crown also known as the ring of fire. The pain was so intense that I felt like my body was going to split in half. I was pushing so hard that sweat was dripping profusely down my entire body. Finally the head came out and Claudia suddenly said. "Amanda, Do Not Push... The umbilical cord is wrapped around the baby's neck!" At this juncture, most people are thinking, "Cord around the neck! That's an emergency and because emergencies like these happen that's why I wanted to have my baby at the hospital to make sure the right medical professionals are there to handle situations like this." But I just listened to what she said and stopped pushing. She quickly and calmly unwrapped the cord and said "Amanda, the cord is fine now and you've got 1 or 2 more pushes." The contraction then came; I pushed and out came my baby girl, Alyssa Isabelle Hess, my pride and joy. But it wasn't over yet. Claudia said, "Amanda, you are hemorrhaging. You are losing too much blood." So she immediately began a uterine massage procedure. The bleeding then stopped. Everyone helped me onto the bed and I held my baby girl for the first time. Claudia and Nicole helped me latch the baby onto my breast to begin the breastfeeding process. We delayed clamping and cutting of the cord to make sure as much of the placental blood could be transferred to the baby to prevent iron deficiency. After about 30 minutes I delivered the placenta and the newborn exam started. Jeremy was so tired at this juncture that he fell asleep with cell phone in hand during the newborn exam. I still make fun of him to this day for falling asleep and I have the picture to prove it! After a little while; however, he soon woke up to make me a bowl of oatmeal with blueberries and strawberries. Soon thereafter, Claudia and Nicole left the house and we snuggled up in bed with our baby girl waiting for the arrival of my mother and grandmother.

To this day, I am so happy with the decision made to have a homebirth. In my heart, I feel that had I gone the mainstream hospital birth road, that augmentation with Pitocin would have occurred due to my lack of progression. During both of my birthing experiences, I never laid down in my bed flat on my back, which is the normal position in a hospital bed. I was always walking around, in the birthing inflatable pool, or on my hands and knees in a squatted position. I can't imagine having to be confined to a hospital bed and unable to move around. I also know from several friends that the hospital doesn't allow you to eat or drink anything during the delivery, no matter how long it may take. I believe this is detrimental to the mother and baby because it could lead to dehydration and lack of energy needed during the birth process. I also gave birth to both of my children in an upright, squatted position that allowed gravity to assist the baby out and the pelvic outlet to expand. I feel certain that had I been in a hospital bed, it would have been very difficult for me to push my babies out. Had I received an epidural and augmentation with Pitocin and then lost feeling due to the paralyzing and numbing effect of epidural anesthesia, which would then result in reliance on a fetal monitor and the nurses to tell me when to push, in addition to the compromising position of the pelvic outlet, I feel that other interventions, such as forceps, vacuum extraction, or episiotomy, would have been necessary.

My first birthing victory was finishing the delivery of Alyssa at 8 pounds, 4 ounces and 21 inches, with no tearing, some blood loss and a small scratch from Alyssa's fingernail as she was coming out. My second birth victory with our son, Gabriel at 8 pounds, 2 ounces and 21 inches, after only three hours of labor, ended with no tearing, no scratches, no blood loss and me taking a 25 minute shower right after the newborn exam and feeling on top of the world! Why can't every woman have this opportunity? Shouldn't every mother be given a choice to make informed decisions for their pregnancy? Wouldn't it be great if birthing started moving in the direction of less medical interventions versus the reality of the past century in which the percent of medical interventions has skyrocketed? Our mission is to give hope to every mother and newborn for a chance at receiving optimal health from the inside out, the way God intended and designed our bodies.

2.
Emerging Emergency

I've always been a numbers type of girl. I sat in the front of the class and I always wanted to be the one who knew the answer. I was the "smart kid." My favorite subject as a child was mathematics, which typically is the nemesis of most kids. My father refers to me as a mathematical genius, in that I never made any grade but an A in math subjects such as geometry, calculus, trigonometry, differential equations and quantitative analysis. As an analytical, numbers-focused person, if the calculations on something make sense, then I understand it and go with it. If the numbers don't make sense, then I start to question it.

There's a story from when I was sixteen years old that my father always likes to tell. I had come home from school to find him sitting at our kitchen table with a slew of papers in front of him, looking stressed out and in despair. This was quite unusual, as I was used to coming home alone because both of my parents worked. I asked him what was going on and he responded, "Amanda, I'm looking at my papers from work. I have been fired and I don't have a job. I'm trying to determine how much money I can earn if I go on straight commission. And will my customers go with me? I think I can earn as much as $60,000 or as little as $18,000. My other option is to take a package worth four months of salary and look for another job, but then I can't contact my current customers." I immediately responded, "Dad, let me look at your numbers." My father said I sat there for 15 minutes studying his production and numbers and then said with confidence and directness,

"Dad, go after them. Do not let your bosses have the business. Go after them, you can do it." To this day, my father refers to this moment as one of the greatest experiences of his life with me. Now, 20 years later, my father continues to work on 100 percent commission and he makes more money in his early 70s than he ever did early in his life.

Now, what does this story have to do with birthing choices?
• Numbers, numbers, numbers.
• Show me the money!

When I became pregnant, the only person I knew on a close, personal basis who had chosen the path of a homebirth was my sister-in-law, Leah. I remember her telling me the unpleasant experience of her first birthing experience in a hospital versus her other two homebirth experiences. All the other women I knew at the time, who were having their babies in the traditional medical model were having episiotomies or Cesareans, or the baby was being pulled out of the womb with forceps or vacuum extraction. I had not heard of or met anybody having a *totally natural, un-medicated* birth in the hospital setting. And, due to my past personal experiences in the hospital, I viewed hospitals as a place to go in case of a medical emergency or significant illness. The mere thought of entering a hospital raises my blood pressure and gives me anxiety. I couldn't imagine trying to give birth in that type of environment. Besides, pregnancy, labor and delivery are not defined in my mind as medical emergencies or illnesses. The process is a completely natural one that God equipped women for. Our society, however, has a very different view on pregnancy and childbirth. My husband and I always joke that once the excitement is over after learning you are pregnant and all the congratulations have been said, pregnancy and childbirth turns into a very different scenario of:

"Congratulations, Mr. and Mrs. Smith! You now have a pathological condition that could result in death. Get ready for the many necessary and questionable/unnecessary procedures and protocols while you are pregnant and in the delivery room!"

Although some of these procedures are necessary and life-saving, the truth is that they should only be used in a very small percentage of situations. Researching these various procedures makes it clearly evident that interventions and unnecessary procedures are overly used in a futile attempt to move women in and out of the hospital as quickly as possible. Cesarean sections are doctor-friendly when it comes to reimbursement, malpractice situations and the doctor's schedule. The amount of interventions used also increases the total cost, test by test or procedure by procedure. So, when analyzing my chances of having a natural birth in a hospital, I felt like the odds were against me. Moreover, after analyzing the cost comparison of having the traditional medical model birth versus a homebirth, it was clear that we would save thousands of dollars in personal and health care costs by having our baby at home.

I remember having a friendly disagreement with a friend who had an induction because she was ready to have the baby, so Mother Nature didn't take its course. After the augmentation with pitocin and the epidural, the doctor "assisted" her by sucking out her son with the vacuum extraction. She didn't think anything was wrong with these procedures, as these were just normal medical protocols to help her have a painless labor and the easiest delivery possible. In my mind, though, the consequences were obvious: every time I talked to her, her son, Zane, was always sick. He seemed to always be on constant antibiotics for chronic ear infections, which finally resulted in ear tube surgery. This was in addition to the chronic allergies and eczema he continually fought against. Zane also had his tonsils and adenoids removed at a very young age. My friend blamed whatever she could, including the daycare, allergy season, or the cold and flu season.

While swimming at our pool one day, he was complaining about his ears due to the water pressure. I thought to myself that this was the perfect opportunity to inquire if she thought his traumatic birth, the multitude of chemicals in the vaccinations, the removal of his first line of immune system defense via his tonsils and adenoids and the constant antibiotics could have affected his immune system and ear function. She retorted, "Absolutely not. I don't know what you're talking about." I told her, "You know that Jeremy and I see a lot of kids in our practice just like Zane and chiropractic could really help him. Don't you think it's about time to think about some other more natural options for him? Aren't you sick and tired of your son being sick?" My friend quickly said, "His pediatrician knows what he is doing and we are going to continue with this path." Needless to say, our opposing viewpoints in health make it difficult to have a close relationship.

I could go on and on with stories of all the women in my life who chose the typical hospital birth setting, with the majority of them ending with an episiotomy or Cesarean. So, after talking with Jeremy, weighing my options and comparing the outcomes and costs of a natural, midwife-assisted childbirth versus a medicated, hospital-assisted childbirth, I chose the path less traveled by women: the homebirth path.

The costs of childbirth can be steep. The charge for an uncomplicated Cesarean section was about $15,800 in 2008. An uncomplicated vaginal birth cost about $9,600, government data shows.[1] The cost can increase depending on how long the patient stays in the hospital and if other complications arise before or after the delivery. The cost of birthing a baby also varies significantly between the insured and the uninsured. Health insurance companies have negotiated contracted fees with doctor and hospital networks and typically charge lower amounts. It is standard protocol for doctors and hospitals to charge almost three times as much for the same procedures to someone who has no insurance.

As noted in the *New York Times* recently, giving birth in the United States is more expensive than any other country in the world. Total costs average $18,329 for a vaginal delivery

---

[1] WedMD

The Cost of Birth

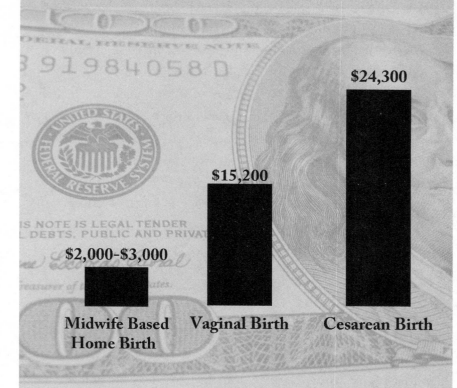

$24,300

$15,200

$2,000-$3,000

Midwife Based Home Birth   Vaginal Birth   Cesarean Birth

The average cesarean birth cost $24,300 in the U.S. last year, compared with $15,200 for a vaginal birth. The average midwife-based home birth costs about $2,000 to $3,000.

-London-based International Federation of Health Plans
http://www.bloomberg.com/news/2012-07-13/aetna-urges
-moms-to-avoid-cesareans-births-to-reduce-risk.html

and $27,866 for a C-section, with the bulk of the bill going to insurers. However, even families with insurance still have to pay about $3,400 out of pocket.[2] Considering that the United States spends more money than anybody else, one would assume that the outcomes would be the best. The disappointing truth, however, is that the U.S. has the highest maternal death rate of any industrialized nation and lags behind 30 developed countries for a mother's well-being, according to a study from Save the Children Humanitarian Organization. The U.S. also has by far the highest first-day death rate in the industrialized world, meaning that more babies die in this country on their first day than all other industrialized countries. These are sad facts when the United States spends $98 billion annually on hospitalization for pregnancy and childbirth.[3]

When I looked into homebirth and found out the cost was $3000, I realized it was quite a difference than hospital birth costs and still less overall, even for those with health insurance. The $3000 included prenatal care, delivery, the birth kit for supplies needed during and after labor and delivery, the pool for the water birth and postpartum care. I spent zero time in the hospital and I stayed in the comforts of my home and bedroom. Immediate recovery time from my first delivery was a couple hours because I felt somewhat weak due to some blood loss during the delivery. There was zero immediate recovery time from my second birth. I had lost no blood, felt great and after the initial nursing of my son, cutting of the cord and release of the placenta, I got out of bed and took a 25-minute shower to clean myself up.

[2] http://www.nytimes.com/2013/07/01/health/american-way-of-birth-costliest-in-the-world.html?hp&_r=2&)

[3] http://www.huffingtonpost.com/2012/08/24/maternal-mortality-rate-infographic_n_1827427.html

The two things that I wanted to avoid at all costs with the delivery of my children were an episiotomy and a Cesarean. Being cut open or scarred for any reason, including the birth of my baby, just didn't sit well with me and for the well being of my baby's neck, spine and brain, I wanted to avoid the use of forceps or vacuum extraction. An episiotomy is an incision performed between the vagina and the rectum that is used to increase the size of the opening of the vagina to assist in delivery of a baby. Cutting from my vagina to rectum just seems barbaric and unnecessary, especially if God gave me a body capable of not only housing a baby for nine months, but also a body capable of delivering a baby.

The following have been reported as side effects of the episiotomy:

- Infection
- Increased pain
- Increase in 3rd and 4th degree vaginal lacerations
- Longer healing times
- Increased discomfort when intercourse is resumed and loss of sexual sensation
- Loss of bladder control
- Greater blood loss during birth
- Severe vaginal tearing that can even lead to fecal incontinence

A WebMD study from August 2005 states that one out of three American women will get episiotomies during childbirth.[4] Some may say that this rate has been declining, which may be

---

4 Web MD 8.26.2005

true; however, with the decline in episiotomies also comes the increase in C-sections over the years. According to a report from the *British Medical Journal*, which studied over 5000 individual births in the United States, the rate of episiotomy with homebirths was found to be 2.1 percent, compared to a rate of over 30 percent with vaginal hospital births.[5] In fact, when I interviewed my midwife, the one question I asked her was, "How many episiotomies have you had to perform in your 25 years of experience?" Her response was, "Many women have had some natural tearing during the delivery, some more than others; however, I have only had to perform a full episiotomy on someone once in my career." It was because of this response that I chose her to be my midwife. I challenge anyone reading this book to ask their obstetrician how many episiotomies he or she has performed during his or her career.

My other fear was the permanent scar, weakened uterine wall and possible adhesions that could be formed should a Cesarean be necessary during my delivery. In a Cesarean, an incision is made through the mother's abdominal wall and uterine wall to get the baby out. There are two types of C-sections: the planned and the unplanned. An unplanned Cesarean is the emergency surgery to save you and your baby because unforeseen complications have occurred during the delivery. What most women don't realize is that the induced, medicated, interventionist approach to birth many times is the direct cause of your baby going into fetal distress and the sudden need for the C-section. Even better, there is the planned C-section, when a mother doesn't want to push her baby out

---

[5] *British Medical Journal*, 6.18.2005

and just schedules the delivery in this way. The modern cheeky term for this is "too posh to push." Women schedule a Cesarean with no medical reason to warrant this surgery.

So, why would a woman need an unplanned C-section? When labor is slow and hard, or stops completely. Interestingly, the increase in inductions through the augmented use of Pitocin and epidural injections can cause the labor to be slow and hard, or to stop altogether. Many times, the act of just entering a hospital can cause a woman's labor to stall or stop completely. She has to hope that the labor gets back on track in a timely manner; otherwise, the hospital protocol will state that the she is not progressing as she should (in other words, not quickly enough for the hospital). Now, it's time to intervene and induce her to speed things up, leading to the myriad of interventions once this is done. Then, with the artificial, stronger contractions caused by the augmentation with pitocin, the baby may become distressed and the heart rate will become irregular. At this point, the woman is most likely medicated, numb, exhausted, starving and dehydrated, so she can't possibly push her baby out by herself. This leads to the unplanned but "save the day" C-section surgery.

Another cause for an unplanned C-section is a potential problem with the placenta or umbilical cord that puts the baby at risk. During the birth of my daughter (my first birth), the cord was wrapped around her neck. I pushed her head out and then heard my midwife say, "Amanda, don't push, don't push right now. The cord is around the baby's neck." Then she calmly and quickly unwrapped the cord from around her neck and proceeded to say, "You can do it, only a little bit left to go. Push!!!" And Alyssa came out. The cord was fine and my midwife placed her on my chest and in my arms to immediately start the bonding and breastfeeding process. Typically the umbilical cord wrapped around the neck is not known until the delivery of a healthy baby and although it may seem scary, this situation is seen in about 2-3 out of 10 normal deliveries.[6] Another umbilical cord concern is cord prolapse; however, this condition is rare. Statistics on cord prolapse vary, but the range is between 0.14 and 0.62 percent of all births. [7]

There are also various conditions of the placenta that may warrant a Cesarean. Placenta previa occurs in some 0.5 percent of pregnant women. Placenta previa is more common in women who have had operations (including a previous C-section) on their womb, or who have a multiple pregnancy. Recently another placenta abnormality known as placenta accreta has increased and seems to also parallel the increasing Cesarean delivery rate. Placenta accreta is a general term used to describe the clinical condition when part of the placenta, or the entire placenta, invades and is inseparable from the uterine wall. An article in the *American Family Physician* reports that 30 percent of reported cases of placenta accreta occur in women with a previous Cesarean.[8] According to the American Pregnancy Association, multiple Cesareans were present in over 60 percent of all cases of placenta accreta.[9] Treatment alternatives vary, depending on the ability of the physician to control blood loss and avoid hemorrhage during and after delivery. The worst-case

---

[6] http://www.babymed.com/labor-delivery/umbilical-cord-around-babys-neck.

[7] http://www.emedicine.com/med/topic3276.htm, http://www.uptodate.com/patients/content/topic. do?topicKey=labordel/2191

[8] http://findarticles.com/p/articles/mi_m3225/is_2_60/ai_55391939

[9] http://americanpregnancy.org/pregnancycomplications/placentaaccreta.html

scenario for placenta accreta included blood transfusions or hysterectomy and resulting loss of the ability to conceive.

In another unplanned C-section scenario, your doctor tells you that your baby is too big to be delivered vaginally and he or she suspects fetal macrosomia. First of all, the diagnosis of fetal macrosomia may be imprecise. For suspected fetal macrosomia, the accuracy of estimated fetal weight using ultrasound biometry is no better than that obtained with clinical palpation. If you believe in a divine, omniscient God, then you should immediately understand that He would not put a baby inside of you that is too big for your body. Have faith in yourself and don't let someone fear you into thinking that you can't deliver your baby. Squatting during the delivery increases the size of the pelvic outlet by as much as ten percent. Of course, lying flat on your back in a hospital bed does not give you the option of squatting and it actually compromises the outlet of the pelvis to expand. The lithotomy position with your feet upright also can cause the mother to attempt to push her baby out against gravity, ascending through the birth canal. Squatting or being upright allows the baby to descend through the birth canal with gravity. A certain percentage of babies are just large in size; however, for some encouragement, as recently reported that in Spain, a woman gave birth to a 13 pound, 11 ounce baby naturally with no epidural.[10]

So, why would you need a planned C-section? The baby may not be in a head-down position close to your due date. The term for this is breech, but if your midwife or obstetrician is aware of this prior to delivery (which they should be), then

---

[10] http://www.huffingtonpost.com/2013/08/08/maria-lorena-13-pound-baby_n_3724688.html

other methods can be used to assist in allowing the baby to get in the best position possible. The common obstetric procedure is called external cephalic version (ECV) performed by your medical doctor with an average success rate of 58percent. This is where the OB will actually try to turn your baby in utero. [11]

There are however ways in which you can work with your body's natural physiology to try and restore balance in your pelvis with the potential of achieving optimal fetal positioning. Maya abdominal massage is one way. Another is the Webster Technique, a specific chiropractic analysis and diversified adjustment to the mother's sacrum. This adjustment helps balance her pelvis and reduce any unnecessary tension to her pelvic ligaments and muscles that may be affecting optimal baby positioning.[12]

Another reason for a planned C-section may be that you are carrying more than one baby (multiples), so we have to schedule you for a C-section. Carrying more than one baby does not automatically mean you have a Cesarean. Many women over the years have had successful vaginal deliveries of multiples.

In another situation, some women might have a condition, such as heart disease, that could be worsened by the stress of labor. In general, women with mild heart disease should attempt childbirth vaginally unless there is another complication that requires a Cesarean section. In fact, some studies indicate that the outcomes are better by having the baby vaginally versus undergoing major surgery. Discuss all options with your providers.[13]

---

[11] American College of Obstetricians and Gynecologists (2000, reaffirmed 2009). External cephalic version. ACOG Practice Bulletin No. 13. Obstetrics and Gynecology, 95(2): 1-7

[12] http://icpa4kids.com/about/webster_technique.htm

[13] http://www.aboutkidshealth.ca/En/ResourceCentres/PregnancyBabies/Pregnancy/MaternalConditionsPregnancy/Pages/Heart-Disease-and-Pregnancy.aspx

Another possibility is that you have an infection that you could pass to the baby during a vaginal birth. Whatever that infection may be, you need to do your due diligence and research it. I personally was positive for Group Beta Strep for both of my pregnancies (also known as GBS positive). The normal hospital protocol would be to immediately hook me up to intravenous antibiotics—during delivery. I knew there had to be an alternative. And sure enough, there were other options. My midwives, Claudia and Debbie, gave me some herbal remedies to administer to protect my baby. And with regards to herpes, the American College of Obstetricians and Gynecologists has recently determined that in women with no active lesions or prodromal symptoms during labor, it is safe to deliver vaginally.[14]

Or, you may have had a C-section before, your doctor says you have the same problems as in an earlier pregnancy and having a VBAC (vaginal birth after Cesarean) could cause uterine rupture. All women should know that the American Pregnancy Association states that 90 percent of women who have had a C-section are eligible for a VBAC. Furthermore, according to the American College of Obstetricians and Gynecologists, a previous C-section with a low transverse incision only has a risk of uterine rupture of 0.2 to 1.5 percent.[15]

There are also some studies that indicate that the induction of labor also increases the rate of uterine rupture. All situations need to be discussed with your health care provider; however, caution is taken if the immediate response by your provider is you are not eligible for a VBAC, with the theory that "once a C-section, always a C-section."

---

[14] http://www.aafp.org/afp/2000/0115/p556.html
[15] http://americanpregnancy.org/labornbirth/vbac.html

The World Health Organization (WHO) recommends that the optimal Cesarean section rate with the best outcomes should be about 5-10 percent. And rates higher than 15 percent seem to do more harm than good.[16]

In 1965, the national U.S. Cesarean rate was in this range at 4.5 percent, but as time went on, we are now at a 32.8 percent rate meaning 1 out of every 3 women now will have a Cesarean section surgery.[17]

This percentage does vary, depending on where you give birth and also who your provider is. During my first pregnancy of 2006 to 2007, the metro Atlanta C-section rates ranged from a low of 22.8 percent at North Fulton Regional to a high of 39.6 percent at Piedmont Hospital.[18]

Considering both of these rates are higher than the WHO recommendation, I was extremely hesitant to walk into a hospital with the hopes of avoiding a Cesarean.

Also, I had to consider some of the possible side effects of having a Cesarean surgery;

- Infection from the incision
- Abdominal adhesions affecting the bladder, bowels and other abdominal organs, which could result in fertility issues for the future. These problems sometimes don't show up until years later.
- Difficulty breastfeeding and bonding with baby
- Increased risk of disease in baby (some studies report that a C-section birth increases a baby's chances of developing asthma, allergies or Type 1 diabetes, because

---

[16] (Althabe and Belizan 2006)

[17] http://www.childbirthconnection.org/article.asp?ck=10456

[18] http://blogginboutbirthandmore.blogspot.com/2008/12/cesarean-rates-atlanta.html

the baby is not exposed to the good bacteria in the
mother's vagina during a normal vaginal birth)
• Placental complications in future pregnancies (as
discussed earlier)

After analyzing the numbers in regards to costs and statistics
of having a baby in the traditional hospital setting, I felt that
a hospital offered me a very low percentage chance of having
birth my way. The odds were stacked against me. Since I am
a normal, healthy, low-risk woman, I didn't want to be just
another statistic of someone who planned their birth one way
and then suffered the fear tactics and intervention measures of
the hospital. In my youth, I had always loved the song "Control"
by Janet Jackson. The lyrics went as follows:

> *This is a story about control, my control*
> *Control of what I say, control of what I do*
> *And this time I'm gonna do it my way*
> *I hope you enjoy this as much as I do*
> *Are we ready? I am? cause it's all about control*
> *And I've got lots of it*
> *When I was 17, I did what people told me*
> *Did what my father said and let my mother mold me*
> *But that was long ago*
> *I'm in control, never gonna stop*
> *Control, to get what I want*
> *Control, I got to have a lot*
> *Control, now I'm all grown up*

That's right, I'm on my own,
I'll call my own shots, thank you

I just wish that more women would get informed and take control of the wonderful gift God has blessed us with: the gift of housing a baby for nine months, the empowerment one receives after birthing their baby naturally, the feeling of being the soul nurturer for the baby for the beginning of life and becoming the ultimate maternal figure God created us to be. The only way to avoid an emerging emergency is to get informed and take control. I know that all birth experiences are different and sometimes even the most planned and thought out births don't always go as expected. I always joke with my husband, Jeremy, that if I could guarantee that all my births went as quickly and easily as my second one with our son, Gabriel, I would have a house full of kids. So… get informed and take control.

Austin's Birth Story
By Leah Hess

Life is all about faith. As believers, we live our lives as a true reflection of the love we have for God. As parents, we are given dominion over our children and it is our deepest calling to make wise and informed decisions. These decisions transcend beyond the day-to-day choices and begin the moment of realization that our bodies, as women, are carrying a precious miracle.

Faith and a desire to seek out the best options for our children guided me and my husband's every step. God blessed us with the opportunity to be parents; our job now was to seek out the best care for our children. We required tremendous faith as we stepped out of the proverbial mainstream medical methods and into a world that made sense, was supported by years of empirical data and allowed the body to reach its potential naturally.

At the moment our first son was born in a prominent hospital in Philadelphia, we were bombarded by choices about how we would care for this beautiful and perfectly formed child. What the medical world deemed as necessary went against every bone in our bodies. As my husband and I questioned these medical doctors and their so-called scientific procedures, it became evident that we were about to enter a lifelong battle in protecting the sanctity of our children's bodies.

Upon leaving the hospital after refusing all "typical medical protocols" and all vaccinations, the Chief of Pediatrics of the hospital informed us that our son would be dead in 2 months' time. His accusations that we were intentionally putting our newborn baby at the risk of death was not exactly what new parents would want to hear. Thankfully, my husband and I agreed on these critical health decisions that *nothing* foreign, *nothing* God didn't create was going to enter this 7 pound, 14 ounce body. First of all, a newborn undergoes tremendous trauma during childbirth. Additionally, our son was born with eczema, which indicated that his immune system was already compromised; therefore, injecting him with foreign and chemically modified ingredients would have only further compromised his body. As I was attempting to rest and recover from the delivery process, my husband stood his ground as he refused the threats and demands of the head pediatrician, which ultimately led to us leaving the hospital one day early to avoid any further confrontation.

Coming from a medical family, the resistance I received from family was imminent. At every family event, the barrage of questions about how we could defy age-old practices loomed over our heads. Our stance continued to be one of free choice. We chose to research the subject of vaccinations and make our own informed decisions. Even 16 years later, my mother still thinks we are foolish and irresponsible, mainly because if she admitted that we were right, it would mean that she made the wrong choice to vaccinate her own children. My husband and I are not trying to make anyone feel they are wrong; we are trying to bring awareness to the subject matter. Is it unreasonable to think doctors don't know everything? Of course not! Many doctors don't even vaccinate their own children. Family, however, is the most difficult to deal with concerning these controversial subjects. Choosing to go down a different path from family members can mean a lonely road.

Our adventure continued as our family moved to Mississippi. One unique thing about Mississippi is that it is one of only two states that have mandatory vaccinations. Just our luck! However, what one person sees as bad luck, I see as an opportunity for change. Our son was only six months old at the time, so we weren't forced with school choices and flying under the radar without vaccinating. Parents wanted desperately to have a choice about whether to vaccinate their children and in 1996, the people of Mississippi did not have that freedom. My husband, being the advocate he is for the freedom of choice, researched court cases and met with individuals who attempted to take on the legal system. He even went as far as to solicit the help of Barbara Loe Fischer with the NVIC (National Vaccination Information Center), who is an advocate for free choice and informed consent and supports families whose children have been injured through vaccinations. Even with the support of the NVIC, the state of Mississippi was not going to change.

As my husband felt the calling to become a chiropractor and attend Life University in Marietta, Georgia, our son was entering preschool. At this point, my husband and I were reading as much as we could about the importance of chiropractic and how God designed the body to heal when nerve system interference is removed and homeostasis returns. Vaccinations still did not play a role in our son's life, but the school was adamant about requiring them. Fortunately, Georgia does have a religious exemption, which satisfied the school. What I wasn't prepared for were the parents. At a prestigious preschool in Atlanta, I didn't expect for parents to confront me with accusations that my child "might give their child a disease." Here were intelligent professionals thinking my child, who never had any foreign toxins injected in his precious body, would give *their* child something—it was preposterous! I simply retorted that if their kids were properly vaccinated against all these diseases they were referring to, then they've got nothing to worry about, since the vaccinations should have totally protected their child from my child. Needless to say, I wasn't welcomed by the majority.

After our horrendous hospital experience with our firstborn, I gave birth to two more children, both born at our home in Marietta, Georgia, in a peaceful and healthy environment with attending midwives. It always perplexes me how majestic and prestigious the hospital was with my first delivery, yet how stressful and fearful I felt there. But during my two home births for my next two children, I was amazed at how peaceful, easy and fearless it was. One of our first calls after our home births was to make an appointment with the chiropractor so our newborn could get evaluated and have a specific chiropractic adjustment if needed. No medical intervention was necessary in either of our homebirths. Now 16 years later, all three of our children are teenagers. None of them have ever received any vaccinations, antibiotics, or pharmaceutical drugs and all three are so much healthier than so many of their friends. We truly believe that our faith in God allowed us to pursue this gratifying, yet lonely, path of health God's way, a path lined with amazing people, two of which are my husband's brother and his wife, Drs. Jeremy and Amanda Hess, who have supported and cared for us in so many ways. We have so much gratitude to God for all He has seen us through!

3.
Fear, Faith and Freedom

When a couple finds out they are expecting, they are filled
with joy and excitement. They start picking out names, dreaming
about what their child will look like and wondering if he or she
will be a boy or a girl. I know when I was pregnant with Alyssa,
I had visions of a blonde-haired, blue-eyed little girl with olive
skin; she'd wear cute bows and pink dresses and play dolls with
me. As it turned out, I did get my little girl with blonde hair,
but with hazel eyes instead. She really doesn't like dresses or
frilly things and refuses to wear hair bows, nor does she like
dolls. Give her a stuffed animal, though and she is thrilled. I
don't really think Jeremy thought about all the details too much,
except that he always kept me well-nourished with healthy
food and prenatal supplements and made sure that I was well-
rested and was in proper alignment through chiropractic care,
so that I would have the best possible pregnancy and labor. Our
mindset was never a mindset of fear, but a mindset that God
gave women the unique structure and ability to house this new
person for nine months, as well as the ability to deliver this
newborn naturally.

But as I progressed in my pregnancy, I discovered that society and even close friends and family members viewed pregnancy very differently. Immediately after their joy and excitement for pregnancy faded, it was apparent that fear began: the fear of prenatal tests, the fear of labor, or the fear of parenting are just a few of the fears people faced. Movies and television often portray pregnancy and labor as a dangerous time in a woman's life that culminates in hours of agonizing labor. Well-meaning family and friends would share their stories of how they would have never made it through labor without an epidural. I remember the conversation when I told my mother I was pregnant. After screaming with excitement, she peppered me with questions: "Amanda, do you know which hospital you're using? What's the name of your obstetrician?" That's when I informed her of our decision to have a homebirth with a midwife and that the obstetrician and hospital were not in our plan unless there were unexpected complications. And since I am a very direct type of individual, I immediately followed with, "And we're not going to do vaccinations." In one five-minute phone call, I had laid it all out on the table. There was a long silence on the phone and since my mother is the opposite of myself (a non-confrontational type of person, a people pleaser and not someone to ever start an argument), she responded, "Amanda, I don't know anything about that, about having your baby at home and about not vaccinating your child. Just do me a favor and don't tell your grandmother. I am here for you for whatever you need."

Some aspects of pregnancy can seem overwhelming and cause anxiety. However the scriptures say that God has not given us a spirit of fear; but of power and of love and of a sound mind. (2 Timothy 2:7) A sound mind is one that is clear and focused on God and His truth. You don't have to be anxious about anything. God's perfect love casts out any fear, including any fear you might have about pregnancy.

Fear in Birth

What causes the spirit of fear in women during labor? An unsupported environment—one filled with bright lights, loud noises, constant conversations and stimulations, restrictions and lack of support—all of which can cause the laboring mother to become startled or fearful. The neocortex, or the thinking part of the brain, becomes stimulated and begins a cycle of fear. To labor most effectively and allow the body to do its work, the neocortex should receive as little stimulation as possible. The laboring woman requires a low-stimuli environment so she can be focused and in a primitive state of mind for the laboring process and culmination of delivery.

The routine use of intravenous needles (IVs), continuous external fetal monitoring (EFM), internal fetal monitoring (IFM) and/or bladder catheters can also cause a spirit of fear. The fluorescent lights in the hospital room, nurses coming and going and constant poking and prodding while hooked up to all sorts of equipment lead to an unsupportive environment. If you are anything like me, you might be afraid of needles. It makes me nervous to have an IV needle in me for many hours. When my friend Charity was in labor with Ethan and had to go to the bathroom, she would have to take the IV and its stand with her. She also had two monitors strapped around her stomach—

one to monitor the strength and frequency of her contractions and the other to monitor how Ethan's heartbeat reacted to the contractions. She later told me how uncomfortable all of it made her and how the straps were attached so tightly that they would dig into her stomach, leaving impressions in her skin. If she tried to move them to get comfortable, they wouldn't pick up the information, which would then alert the nurse sitting at her desk in the lobby. She would come in and fix the monitors, all the while scolding Charity for moving them. I was shocked when Charity said she was scolded and yelled at while in labor. She was told to lie there and be still. As she laid there watching the monitor, waiting to hear Ethan's next heartbeat, she said she felt completely overwhelmed. After she was given an epidural, she had to have a bladder catheter inserted and because she was completely paralyzed from the waist down, she would not be able to get up and go to the restroom anymore. She wasn't even allowed to eat or drink; she was only allowed to have ice chips to moisten her mouth. As she described it to me, "I was officially a prisoner in my hospital bed."

While she recapped her experience to me, I had to inform her that my birth with Alyssa at my house in my own bedroom was quite the opposite experience. I was allowed to move around, sit up, lie down, walk around and do whatever I wanted to do while laboring. I could get in my pool of warm water if I wanted to, or I could get out if I needed to do so. I could go to the bathroom whenever I needed to and Jeremy was there the whole time giving me water and juice to keep me hydrated. I told her that I didn't want anything to eat during my labor because I thought for sure that I was going to vomit since I kept burping up the taste of lasagna from dinner that evening. Jeremy still jokes that the whole experience seemed like I went into this other state of mind. I started to moan, groan and hum, making noises that he had never heard before. I wanted the lights to be very dim and no one to be talking. The room was completely silent. Claudia, my midwife and Nicole, her apprentice were there, but I really don't remember them being there and saying much to me until it was time to push and assist me as Alyssa crowned and was born.

With Charity's first pregnancy with Ethan, she viewed labor pains as unnecessary, since everybody has an epidural and comes out of the hospital just fine. She thought having an epidural would give her the best labor possible because it was an "easy" way out; however, the opposite was true. God created pain in labor to assist the birthing woman to be able to feel when to push the baby out of the birth canal. Charity was blinded by the fear of pain in labor and as it turned out, Ethan's birth was her worst birthing experience. She looks back now and says how ironic it is that society and the medical field shun a pregnant woman if she is seen smoking, drinking alcohol, or taking drugs, because of the effects all these artificial stimulants could have on the baby; however, everything changes once the pregnant woman enters the hospital for labor. Once you are in the hospital, you can have drugs and lots of them. Charity says that she didn't acknowledge that all the drugs had the potential to hurt her and Ethan and the routine procedures only caused fear and made her birth more difficult. Fear gives false evidence for things that appear to be real; it keeps you from acknowledging the truth; and it leaves you uncertain, unsafe, unsupported and anxious. Fear causes us to make decisions we would not usually make. Pregnant women are told to never take a single drug. Charity was told that nothing was safe to take while pregnant, though during labor, the rules changed and she could have many drugs. After delivering Ethan, she was ashamed that she allowed the hospital staff to give her fourteen different drugs. She was shocked that this was normal procedure. She was told that the medicine in epidurals is localized to the spine and does not cross the placenta to the baby. The consent form she signed never mentioned possible side effects for her baby. In light of all this, she felt justified in her pursuit of a pain-free delivery.

When Ethan was two years old Charity ran in a 5K race in support of her friend Joan, a breast cancer survivor. When she first started training, she feared that she wouldn't be able to run the entire three miles. She feared her legs would give out and she wouldn't finish. But she kept training, eating healthy and nutritious foods and received regular chiropractic care so she would be in the best shape possible for the race. The big day of the race finally came. She started out slowly, pacing herself and she at first thought that it was going to be easy. But the road was much steeper than the road she had trained on and as she continued running, it gradually got more difficult. She started to get tired and her muscles started to burn and ache. Near the end she got discouraged and wanted to give up. She literally wanted to run away and not finish. She felt as though she couldn't run the last mile. She remembers telling herself, "Keep fighting, you are almost there! You have been training for this for months, don't give up now, you can do this—just keep pressing on!" When she renewed her mind with the truth, it helped her to have faith in her body's ability and all the training she had done to get to this point. It was tough, but she kept pushing through step by step. Finally she reached the finish line and in her words, "I felt amazing and free. I had made it! I had persevered!"

Many women experience these same types of fearful feelings during labor. These negative feelings come from your intellectual mindset, the neocortex and result in fear. During labor, however, the neocortex is supposed to be at rest so that primitive brain structures can more easily release the necessary hormones during this critical time for mother and baby. Fear also causes your labor to stall. If you are fearful in early labor your body may release catecholamines or adrenaline (a stress hormone) that causes physiological responses in direct opposition to what the body requires during labor. These "stress responses" may increase your heart rate and respiration and decrease the blood flow to the uterus. This results in tension, muscle soreness and fatigue, increased pain and a less effective labor. Most of the time, these fear responses are felt during times of transition.

Charity experienced them during the natural birth of her second child, Lauren. During the transition period of Lauren's birth, she was sitting up in her bed pushing. Her husband was on the left of her and her mother was on the right. She had been pushing for 20 or 30 minutes at this point and she started to have flashbacks of Ethan's birth in the hospital and how she pushed for three and a half hours and ended up with a level four episiotomy. She thought to herself, "I had all the experts there to help me with Ethan. I couldn't do it then. For sure there is no way I can do this now, naturally, with just my husband, mother and a midwife here." These thoughts caused Charity to become fearful. She says she started to scream and freak out. She remembers yelling at her midwife, Claudia, "She is never going come out!" Claudia immediately responded in her usual calm and soothing voice, "Charity, you need to stop screaming. Calm down, relax and focus. Every time you push with a contraction, her head will come out a little and pull back and push out a little and pull back, eventually pushing the baby all the way out." During this critical part of Lauren's birth, Claudia also continued to massage and stretch Charity's perineum with olive oil to prevent tearing. This natural protocol was never offered at the hospital with her previous birth with Ethan. Several minutes then went by when Claudia said, "Charity, I can feel her head. Reach down and feel it." Charity says she placed her hand in the birth canal and could feel a head full of hair. It was a moment that she will never forget. It gave her that little bit of faith that she could persevere and finish that race. As Lauren began to crown, Charity's pelvic floor began to burn. Some women may think burning is abnormal. Pain they understand, but burning not so much. But Charity had read about this burning sensation, also known as the "ring of fire." Just like when our legs burn while running, this burning sensation meant the finish line was in sight. Lauren was about to be born. All Charity needed to do was push through to the very end. This "ring of fire" wasn't a detriment, but an encouragement. It was a sign her body was doing exactly what God had gifted it to do. At this point, Claudia lovingly suggested Charity get up again and try pushing on the birthing stool. With her husband behind her helping to support her body, Charity was able to push out Lauren within ten minutes. Her total delivery from start to finish was only three and a half hours.

The term "pain in labor" has a negative connotation in society. What most people don't know is the word "pain" and the word "toil" are actually the same Hebrew word *etzev*, meaning toil, distress, labor and trouble. God uses the word *etzev* throughout the Bible, but it never conveys the meaning of pain. Unbearable pain does not always accompany childbirth. To labor and to toil indicates hard work. Hard work appropriately describes the strenuous labor involved in giving birth (in the case of the woman) and the labor involved in plowing, digging, ripping and sowing the land (in the case of the man). This is better known as the curse of Adam and Eve after sinning in the Garden. Over the years, man has invented many labor-saving machines to lighten his workload of farming the ground, but society has done the exact opposite for women. Instead, it has multiplied in her mind suggestions of fear from countless sources, both ancient and modern, thus making her labor indefinitely harder than need be. Just as men have to work the land to produce food, a woman has to work with her body to bear a child. Both types of work can cause aches and pains in our muscles; however, the bearing of children is one of the most wonderful and joyous experiences of a woman's life.

Pain is the most common reason for a physical consultation with a doctor in the United States.[1] It is defined as an unpleasant sensation occurring in varying degrees of severity

[1] Debono, DJ; Hoeksema, LJ; Hobbs, RD (August 2013). "Caring for Patients with Chronic Pain: Pearls and Pitfalls". Journal of the American Osteopathic Association 113(8): 620–627. doi:10.7556/jaoa.2013.023. PMID 23918913.

as a consequence of illness or injury. This is how many health care providers view pregnancy. They believe a woman's body is not built to withstand the process of giving birth naturally and they believe that pain-relieving drugs help women emotionally and physically cope, with the potentially false belief system that the act of giving birth is a life-threatening event. Pregnancy, however, is not an illness or an injury. A woman's body is not broken; it is designed to give birth. God has given all women the power and strength to give birth naturally. Society and other principalities are hard at work deceiving pregnant women and their families. They multiply the thoughts of fear in every woman's heart. Through artificial pharmaceuticals, women get false promises to avoid the pain, work and toil associated with childbirth.

It has been six years since my birthing victory with Alyssa and three years since my second one with Gabriel. Being a woman in this "natural birthing" category and on top of that a chiropractor, puts me in the minority of the minorities. Some of the statements I have heard over the years are:

"Childbirth doesn't have to be painful. I don't have to suffer. I can get this epidural and not feel a thing. I can just lie there and the experts can also speed this up with Cervidil and Pitocin. Then I can be relaxed and go home the next day with my baby. Everybody else I know did it this way, so it must be okay. Why would anyone choose to suffer through hours of agonizing pain? A woman like yourself who wants to have natural childbirth must be crazy. I could never do that. My pain tolerance is too low. What if something bad happens? My baby could die or

I could die. I would never take the chance of having my baby outside a hospital setting."

When a woman says these kinds of things to me, I feel sorry for her. I feel most sorry about her misguided fear with pregnancy and labor and it distresses me that women have lost any type of empowerment and self-confidence in themselves and the gift of childbearing from God.

The justifications for induction also shock myself and my husband:

"My mother is scheduled to fly into town on Saturday to help me with the baby for a couple of weeks, so if the baby doesn't come soon, then we are going to induce. She only has so much time off from work, so she can't be sitting here for a week or whatever waiting for my baby to arrive."

Or:

"The baby is due December 26. I already talked to my OB and he said it was perfectly fine to schedule the induction on the 20th. He's going on vacation on the 23rd, so it works out great for both of us. That way, the baby will be here for Christmas and it won't mess up Christmas for my other kids too."

The Christmas story above ended with an induction on December 20th. When the pregnant mother entered the hospital, she wasn't dilated at all. After all the induction drugs were administered and labor continued to not progress as it should have (to the surprise of everyone), she had a Cesarean. I desperately wanted to say to her that her baby wasn't ready to be born yet. It's no wonder her labor didn't progress; her body wasn't ready. She should have waited for her body's innate physiological response to take it course, but I didn't say any of that. Instead, I congratulated her on her new baby and was thrilled she brought the child into my office for his first chiropractic adjustment. She, however, was too sore from the Cesarean and wanted to wait a couple of weeks before she got her chiropractic adjustment.

The scriptures say, "When a woman gives birth to a baby, she has pain, because her time has come. But when her baby is born, she forgets the pain, because she is so happy that a child has been born into the world (John 16:21)." The innate wisdom of the body uses pain as a signal to a woman that the baby is coming soon, which motivates mothers to get up, move around and change positions to alleviate some of the pain. In active labor, contractions last an average of 60 seconds. Your body and the baby are given breaks in between contractions and the pain is not continuous. God designed it this way to have pain serve its purpose.

Fear is strong, but faith is stronger. Through faith and increased knowledge, we can overcome and conquer our fears about pregnancy and labor. Fear is not from God. Just the contrary, in fact: God wants you to have faith in His power and strength. You can have a spirit of faith by trusting that God has designed your body for the purpose of birth and the innate wisdom to know exactly what to do. This faith will help you stay calm and confident during labor, giving you a peace and security.

Faith is the opposite of fear. Faith is confidence in what we hope for and assurance about what we do not see (Hebrews 11:1). Although we cannot see our ligaments and muscles working inside our body during pregnancy and labor, we have faith they are going to do their job. God gave our bodies an innate intelligence that regulates everything inside of us, this intelligence creates special hormones to help a woman during labor: the "love" hormone, called oxytocin; the "feel good" hormones, called endorphins; and the "fight or flight" hormones, called adrenaline. These hormones are steadily produced in un-medicated births.[2] Oxytocin stimulates powerful contractions, which help to thin and open (dilate) the cervix, move the baby down and out of the birth canal, expel the placenta and limit bleeding at the site of the placenta. Endorphins are calming and pain-relieving hormones produced in response to stress and pain. Adrenaline hormones ensure survival and high levels are produced if a women feels threatened or fearful. Oxytocin and endorphins are released when a women feels safe, calm and confident. The result is relaxation, confidence and decreased pain. Though they cannot be seen, all of these hormones play a big part in regulating the process of labor and birth.

One of the purposes of a woman is to reproduce. Pregnancy and childbirth are gifts to women; men will never be able to experience the feeling of a baby growing and moving inside their body. Many pregnancy and birth books describe labor contractions as waves that come to peak and then slowly taper off. Women should trust and have faith in the purpose of each contraction. If you work against them, your body will tense up, causing your labor to stall and the contractions to be painful. When you relax and let the waves of contractions wash over you, the muscles around the pelvis will loosen and relax, opening

[2] Childbirth Connection

the cervix. Contractions are a blessing. They cause the baby to move and turn little by little, working with your body for good. They will produce a miracle, a baby, God's special gift. I don't believe God designed birth as a time of suffering. I do believe that God's mercies are new every morning. He is merciful even during one of the most physically demanding times in a woman's life. Not only is He merciful, but He is also faithful—faithful in designing and equipping you to conceive and bear children. He will also be faithful in giving you strength and perseverance by helping you push through each contraction. My faith increased with my labor and delivery of each of my children. At times, childbirth and parenting feels like a trial, but through every trial, you become a stronger individual and develop a deeper faith and trust in how God designed you. Faith and trust produce freedom.

Freedom in Birth

While Charity was pregnant with Ethan, her ignorance and lack of understanding about how God created a woman's body to birth naturally, caused her to be defiant to natural methods and be blinded to the truth. She wouldn't listen when her mother mentioned anything about birthing naturally and that the drugs given to her would also affect her baby. After Ethan's birth, she realized everything her mother said was true. Every drug and every intervention really did affect him. She realizes now that it isn't normal for all these newborns to go into fetal distress and it isn't normal for this many women to have episiotomies and Cesarean surgeries. She is saddened now looking back at her son's traumatic birth. However, through that experience, she

Preterm Births

Preterm Birth is the Birth of an Infant Prior to 37 Weeks of Pregnancy

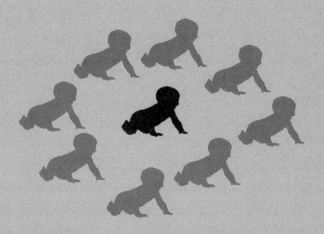

1 out of 9 Infants Born in the United States are Preterm

Preterm births have increased 36% since the early 1980's.

became knowledgeable and took back the false belief system that women aren't equipped to birth naturally. She changed the way she thought about her body and her body's innate ability to birth.

Many parents go into pregnancy and birth without any research, knowledge, or classes, all of which could help them make informed decisions. Society places all their trust in doctors and protocols, but in our opinion, placing our trust there and not in what God has given us has led us to a place of embarrassment when compared to the rest of the world.

It's no wonder that :

1. The pre-term birthrate has risen 36 percent since the early 1980s. This means that 1 out of every 9 infants born in the United States is pre-term, meaning that they were born prior to 37 weeks of pregnancy.

2. In 2006, according to the U.S. Centers for Disease Control and Prevention, more than 1 in 5 births in the United States was induced. This rate more than doubled from 1990.

3. Induction of labor for non-recognized indications is associated with a 67 percent increased relative risk of Cesarean section (compared with spontaneous labor).

4. Induction also significantly increases the chance of the infant requiring Neonatal Intensive Care Unit nursery care (an increased relative risk of 64 percent) or other treatment (an increased relative risk of 44 percent) when compared with the spontaneous labor onset.[3]

[3] Rosalie M. Grivell, Aimee J. Reilly, Helena Oakey, Annabelle Chan, Jodie M. Dodd. Maternal and neonatal outcomes following induction of labor: a cohort study. Acta Obstetricia et Gynecologica Scandinavica, 2012; 91 (2): 198 DOI: 10.1111/j.1600-0412.2011.01298.x

Induced Births
The Risks behind Augmenting your Labor

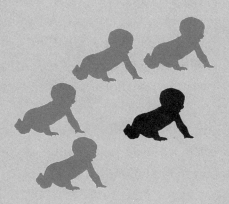

In 2006, according to the U.S. Centers for Disease Control and Prevention, more than 1 in 5 births in the United States were induced. This rate more than doubled from 1990.

Induction of labor for non-recognized indications area associated with a 67% increased relative risk of cesarean section (compared with spontaneous labor). It also significantly increased the chance of the infant requiring Neonatal Intensive Care Unit nursery care (an increased relative risk of 64%) or treatment (an increased relative risk of 44%) when compared with the spontaneous labor onset.

-Rosalie M. Grivell, Aimee J. Reilly, Helena Oakey, Annabelle Chan, Jodie M. Dodd. Maternal and neonatal outcomes following induction of labor: a cohort study. Acta Obstetricia et Gynecologica Scandinavica, 2012; 91 (2): 198 DOI: 10.1111/j.1600-0412.2011.01298.x

5. The World Health Organization recommendations of optimal rates of Cesarean section—only 5 to 10 percent—have the best outcomes for women and babies. Rates above 15 percent seem to do more harm than good.[4]

6. In 1965, when it was first measured, the national U.S. Cesarean section rate was near this optimal rate, at 4.5 percent. However, the national Cesarean section rate is now much higher.[5] After steeply increasing over more than a decade, it leveled off at 32.8 percent in 2010 and 2011[6]. **In other words, 1 in 3 women are now having major surgery to birth their baby.**

7. The average Cesarean birth cost $24,300 in the United States last year, compared with $15,200 for a vaginal birth, according to the London-based International Federation of Health Plans. [7]

8. Daily NICU costs exceed $3,500 per infant and it is not unusual for costs to top $1 million for a prolonged stay.

9. Childbirth practices researcher Katherine Hartmann, MD, Ph.D, estimates that close to 1 million unnecessary episiotomies are performed in the U.S. each year. A third of American women get episiotomies during childbirth.[8]

10. Americans "are living longer, sicker" with more chronic illness, says Reed Tuckson of the United Health Foundation.[9]

[4] (Althabe and Belizan 2006)
[5] (Taffel et al. 1987)
[6] Hamilton et al. 2012
[7] http://www.bloomberg.com/news/2012-07-13/aetna-urges-moms-to-avoid-cesareans-births-to-reduce-risk.html
[8] http://www.webmd.com/baby/guide/delivery-methods
[9] http://www.usatoday.com/story/news/nation/2012/12/10/health-rankings-states/1759299/

11. The United States has by far the highest first-day death rate in the industrialized world. It ranks 41st in child well being.[10]

12. The United States spends $98 billion annually on hospitalization for pregnancy and childbirth, but the U.S. maternal mortality rate has doubled in the past 25 years. The U.S. ranks 50th in the world for maternal mortality, meaning 49 countries were better at keeping new mothers alive.[11]

On the natural birth road, the statistics paint a very different picture:

1. In 1900, almost all babies in the U.S. were born at home. In 1940, 44 percent of births still took place at home, but by 1969, that figure was 1 percent. Physicians and hospitals had taken over the task of helping mothers give birth. That percentage slightly dipped through the 1980s and home births are still rare, with less than 1 percent of babies born at home.[12]

2. The UK's National Institute for Health and Clinical Excellence (NICE) report concluded that women who give birth at home are more likely to deliver vaginally and to have greater satisfaction from the experience, when compared with women who plan to give birth in a hospital.[13]

[10] Save the Children Humanitarian Organization
[11] http://www.huffingtonpost.com/2012/08/24/maternal-mortality-rate-infographic_n_1827427.html
[12] http://www.cdc.gov/nchs/data/databriefs/db84.pdf
[13] http://en.wikipedia.org/wiki/National_Institute_for_Health_and_Clinical_Excellence

3. In North America, a 2005 study found "similar mortality rates for low-risk hospital births and planned home births." The study found that mothers who gave birth at home were less likely to require medical interventions like a Cesarean section or forceps delivery. About 12 percent of women intending to give birth at home needed to be transferred to the hospital.[14]

4. The average midwife-based home birth costs about $2,000 to $3,000.

5. A study in the *British Medical Journal*, which was based on nearly 5,500 home births involving certified professional midwives in the United States and Canada and considered one of the largest studies for home births, showed 88 percent had positive outcomes, while 12 percent of the women were transferred to hospitals, including 9 percent for preventive reasons and 3 percent for emergencies. The study showed an infant mortality rate of 2 out of every 1,000 births, about the same as in hospitals at the time.[15]

6. Mothers themselves had fewer medical interventions like epidurals for pain or fetal monitoring in the homebirths. No maternal deaths at home were reported in the analysis. In fact, mothers did better with fewer medical procedures, as they were less likely to suffer lacerations and infections.[16]

7. A large 2009 study reported that in the Netherlands, a planned homebirth led by a midwife at onset of labor

[14] http://www.bmj.com/content/330/7505/1416

[15] http://www.utsandiego.com/news/2011/jul/05/home-birth-on-the-rise-by-a-dramatic-20-percent/all/?print

[16] (Taffel et al. 1987)

"does not increase the risks of perinatal mortality and severe perinatal morbidity among low-risk women, provided the maternity care system facilitates this choice through the availability of well-trained midwives and through a good transportation and referral system.[17]"

Through educating and empowering yourself, you, along with all parents, can make the best-informed decisions for your children, health and lives. When you walk in understanding and truth, you will have freedom and power. You are the best advocate possible of your body, your birth and your baby. The decisions you make, whether informed or uninformed, will define who you are and how your life experiences will be.

[17] http://www.ncbi.nlm.nih.gov/pubmed/19624439

Chandler's Birth Story

By Crystal Nutt

In December 2011, my husband, David and I found out we were pregnant with our first child. I had always planned to have a routine hospital birth with an epidural because that's just what most people seem to do. Birth looked incredibly painful in any movie I'd ever seen, and I never really questioned the hospital birth process or understood why anyone would ever go natural. I wasn't trying to be a hero, that sounded like a lot of pain and I didn't see why it was necessary. So, I found a doctor's office that I liked and began my prenatal care. Shortly after, we learned we were going to have a precious baby boy.

A few months into my pregnancy, I started going to a chiropractor. For our introductory meeting, Dr. Amanda Hess talked about her homebirth experiences. What she shared caused me to completely change my birth plan. She said that epidurals made pushes during labor ineffective. I later learned that when the baby is medicated, it is also harder for him to do his job of spinning through the pelvis to come out.

Inductions and epidurals counteract the body's natural capabilities to proceed with the birth process, which can slow down labor and make it more difficult. What scared me was learning that these routine hospital interventions can lead to more interventions, like a forceps or vacuum extraction delivery, both of which put a lot of strain on baby's neck, (leading to further problems), or worse, a C-section. And other than my baby being harmed or dying during childbirth, a C-section was my worst fear.

So from that point on, I decided I could no longer risk having an epidural. I now knew too much! However, I also knew that I couldn't possibly swing a non-medicated birth without more information. So, I talked with two friends whom I knew advocated natural birth and they both suggested the Bradley Method. Within a couple of weeks of my non-epidural decision, my husband and I were committed to a 12-week Bradley class.

In addition to the class, I read several books pertaining to natural birth and watched Ricki Lake's exposé on birth in America, *The Business of Being Born*. Everything I read and saw confirmed what I'd learned from my chiropractor. Plus, my mom had me naturally, although it was not planned that way. Since she passed away almost ten years ago, I felt like this was a way I could identify with her. I knew if she could do it I could, too.

In all of that reading, I learned two more interesting things. The first was that medicated babies can have a harder time latching on to nurse for a few hours after birth; this was more incentive for me to go natural. The second was that in order for labor to progress, you have to be relaxed. I knew that I personally could not possibly be relaxed in a hospital. I also had the feeling that if I knew an epidural was available when it got tough, I might change my mind and get one.

I needed to put myself in a situation where pain meds were not available, barring an emergency, of course. After much discussion with my husband, research, interviews with midwives and previous homebirthers, prayer and an unsuccessful search for a local birthing center, we decided to attempt a homebirth using licensed professional midwife, Charlotte Sanchez, her assistant Rachel and doula Chasery Baxter. We did dual care with Charlotte and the doctor's office for a while. I then decided to see only Charlotte. She was much more confident in the ability of a healthy, low-risk woman's body to handle labor and birth naturally.

Now, I'll fast forward to the labor and birth part of my story. September 7th, which was my due date, came and went, 41 weeks came and went and then finally, late one night at 41½ weeks, I decided to start taking herbs to kick start labor. After only one dose, I started having contractions. I called Charlotte at about midnight to let her know what was going on and she said to let her know when they were around seven minutes apart. They never got to seven minutes apart that night, but I did have a contraction every ten to twenty minutes. I managed to sleep between them since I knew I'd need my energy. That went on all night until about 8 or 9 am.

That morning I called Chasery and told her to go ahead and make the hour trip to my house—labor had started! Then I got in the shower and labor stopped! After updating Chas and Charlotte, we decided I should take more herbs to get labor going again. Chasery arrived and she began giving me the herbs and trying out some reflexology. While we were waiting for labor to start, David began filling up the birthing pool for my dream waterbirth. I'd heard it would take the edge off of contractions.

Time was passing and labor hadn't really started hard yet, so that afternoon Charlotte said I could try castor oil. I did not want to do that, but she assured me that if I took it with ice cream and not the acidic orange juice (which most people took it with), it wouldn't be that bad. I was ready to have my baby today and not tomorrow, so Chas mixed it up, I took it and not more than an hour later I threw up. I was in labor again!

I really don't remember much before transition except that I sat on the birthing ball and rocked for a little while. I remember going to my bathroom and leaning over the counter as contractions got stronger. Chasery brought a rebozo and tied it around my hips to alleviate some pain.

Yet, as contractions got stronger, I wanted to be touched less and less. Chasery finally suggested I get in the shower. I love hot showers, so that sounded wonderful. With my pregnant belly, I sat down in my stall shower and turned the water on as hot as I could stand. It was so relaxing. I was in transition then and the contractions were the hardest of the entire labor.

As I mentioned earlier, I knew that I was supposed to relax my whole body during contractions, so I attempted to do this during the tough ones by moaning and counting. I knew that once I got to between 30 and 60, the worst was over. The funniest part is that during some of those shower contractions, I sang to myself "Soft Kitty" from The Big Bang Theory. No scripture or worshipful songs came to mind. Oh, no, but "Soft Kitty" did. So much for a spiritual moment!

While I was in the shower, Charlotte arrived. I got out for her to check me and we were all so excited that I was dilated to 7. I had no concept of time, but it must have been around 7 pm at that point. Back to the shower I went for more moaning and groaning. Meanwhile, my husband's job was to coach and encourage me during labor. He did a wonderful job, except for one little blip. I remember him sitting outside the shower in a folding chair playing on his iPod, of all things. My contractions were getting pretty close together and I counted and moaned through four hard ones in a row with no break. When those were over, I parted the shower curtain and said, "David, I just had 4 contractions in a row. I could use some encouragement here!" He looked up from his iPod and said (in a monotone voice), "Oh yeah, you're doing a good job." He really was a great coach, though.

After 10 to 20 minutes, I got out of the shower and Charlotte checked me again: I was still at 7. I stayed out this time and just lay in my bed. The contractions were the strongest at this point and I just whimpered uncontrollably until I dilated to 10. Chasery was so encouraging and Charlotte watched in silent support from the foot of the bed.

The next thing I remember, Charlotte asked if I wanted to get in the tub to have my waterbirth. I sure didn't feel like walking from the bedroom to the breakfast area, but I did. I got in and it felt so good. It really did take the edge off. That was around 8:30 pm. At that point, I remembered it was time to put in the lasagna (Charlotte had cleverly suggested earlier that I make one ahead and freeze it). We all laughed at the fact that I wasn't too busy to forget.

Rachel got there just in time for me to say, "I feel like I gotta poop!" We all knew what that meant—it was time to push! Charlotte suggested I get on my knees and hang my head and arms over the side of the pool. David was sitting on a cushioned bench in front, where my head was. This was the point that I was thankful we'd taken a class, because we had practiced pushing. David was the most helpful during that time. He held my hands as I bore down and pulled away with all my might and then he leaned back and pulled my arms to give me some leverage. It felt good to push, yet painful at the same time.

Finally, after I'd been pushing a little while, I started to feel the baby move down. Charlotte told me to reach down and feel his head, so I did. That was such an incredible moment. We were finally about to meet our son. It was so exciting! Plus, I was almost done with the pain, which made me want to push even harder because I wanted him out. I pushed a few more times and continued to feel him come further down and then slip a little back up after each push. It was just a little frustrating, even though I'd been taught that was supposed to happen.

I continued pushing and felt his head a couple more times and he was coming further out. Charlotte warned me ahead of time that whenever the head came out, I should stop pushing so she could check for the cord. I remember those last two pushes; I pushed with everything I had and I even heard myself grunt like an animal—I couldn't control it. Then I felt a pop and his head was out. Charlotte instructed me not to push. That little boy was in the caul, as my water never broke.

Although I didn't really know what was going on then, I found out later that the cord was wrapped around his neck twice and he was unconscious. Charlotte broke my water and unwrapped the cord, then I pushed the rest of his body out. I flipped over and Charlotte took him and instructed her team, "Cut the cord, cut the cord!" A few silent moments passed as we watched Charlotte give him mouth-to-mouth and waited for him to breathe. I said the quickest prayer: "Lord, please don't let my baby die after all this." Then I was holding him and she gave him a couple of chest compressions. The birth team told me to rub and talk to him, so I did. Finally, I heard him take in a little breath, then I heard a tiny whimper, followed by a slightly louder one. What a wonderful relief—our sweet baby was okay.

That was the beginning of celebration time, although I still had to birth the placenta. I nursed that sweet baby within about ten minutes of his birth to help the placenta detach and soon after that I felt ready to push again. I pushed and Charlotte tugged slightly and the placenta was out. After that, Rachel and Chasery helped me out of the tub and straight to my bathroom for a victory shower while they checked, weighed and measured my darling baby boy.

Charlotte then gave me a thorough stitch job, since my son came out with his hand up by his head. She later told me she really took her time on me, because she knew I was kind of stubborn about constantly working out and she didn't want me further damaging myself. Then, it was time for the lasagna.

It was all so wonderful. I was so glad to be finished and to have done it naturally. After he came to, my baby was so alert and was such a super nurser. My little boy, however, did not receive his name until the next day, as my husband and I were too indecisive. The day after he was born, we decided to call him Chandler David. He's absolutely precious.

I'm blessed to have been able to have the labor and birth of my dreams in my own home. I know it doesn't always go as planned. I'm thankful that almost everything went well and that Charlotte was so wonderful for the part that didn't. The health and safety of my baby was worth it. I would do it again the same way. Thank you so much for taking the time to read my story. Many blessings.

4.
Artificial, Processed
& Preserved Children

Fast Food Generation

My wife and I are both principled, specific chiropractors and have one of the busiest chiropractic practices in the world. We watch less than ten hours of network TV programming per year and we make it a habit not to follow current events. We don't vaccinate our children. Neither of us has taken any prescription or over-the-counter medications in over a decade and our children have never had any antibiotics, pills, shots... nothing. On top of that, we don't eat fast food. Our children have had fast food fewer times than the fingers on one hand and only because they weren't under our supervision. Our daughter, Alyssa, calls Ronald McDonald a "tricky" clown who tricks kids into thinking his food is good and healthy for kids by giving them toys and having playlands at his restaurant. Some parents are proud of different things about their children and we like to brag about the fact that a McDonald's French fry has yet to cross their lips!

When our kids were babies, Amanda nursed Alyssa until she was 22 months old and Gabriel until he was 26 months old. We started making food for them at about 6 months old as a supplement to breastfeeding and we knew exactly what was in the food they were eating. We bought fresh, organic fruits and vegetables as much as we could. We wanted to avoid food, snacks and canned baby food tainted with pesticides, chemicals and preservatives. It doesn't take a genius to realize that fresh food is perishable where as canned baby food has a "shelf life" of approximately 2 years. What people may not realize is that fresh baby food is so easy to prepare and freeze for future use. We would typically make six to eight trays of various foods on Sunday evening in preparation for the week. The key word here is preparation. We've heard it said that in life, you are either "preparing or repairing". The same goes with our babies; either we prepare properly to get educated on topics such as health and natural foods, or we end up repairing the damage that has been done by not knowing the correct methods of rearing up our kids naturally, the way we believe God intended.

Maybe it's just us, but everywhere we turn we see "junk food" (at least, that's what we used to call it when we were growing up). When our daughter was in preschool, we were shocked (and still are) at the amount of processed and fast food that the school served to the 2- and 3-year-olds. On any given week in her class, there were cookies on Monday brought by a caring grandma, McDonald's on Wednesday supplied by the preschool, Dunkin' Donuts on Thursdays gifted by a loving classmate's mother and Friday would round out the week with a big cookie cake for a classmate's birthday. Oh and don't forget about special days and holiday weeks. The excessive amount of sugar is unbelievable, a rollercoaster through each proceeding holiday. There's gobs and gobs of candy, cakes and cookies beginning with Halloween, the school's fall carnival, Grandparents' Day, Thanksgiving feasts, Christmas and holiday celebrations, Valentine's Day, Easter, spring carnivals, end of the year school parties and we could go on and on. Our children just recently celebrated Dads and Donuts for the morning, as well as a Moms and Muffins party. On each occasion, Amanda prepared an organic snack the night before so our kids could still participate and have fun with us.

One particular holiday that we loathe is Halloween. Yes, it is fun for the kids to dress up as princesses and superheroes, but the sheer amount of junk consumed is astronomical! Children's Healthcare of Atlanta states that at Halloween, the average child will consume up to three cups of sugar—the equivalent to 200 packets' worth—and gain 2.2 pounds. And while all parents attempt to ration out the Halloween spoils over time, imagine your child consuming 30 packets of sugar daily for seven days straight. It never fails that every year after Halloween, kids show up in our chiropractic office with fever, colds and compromised immune systems. We wonder if parents even put the puzzle pieces together that refined sugars and sugar in general are known to suppress the immune system, promote inflammation and outright make us sick. The kids end up being "sick and symptomatic" and out of school at that time of the year and pharmaceuticals get ushered onto the scene as the medical community touts over-the-counter medications, antibiotics and flu shots as the saving grace. The truth is that God gave the body the ability to heal itself, even after the onslaught of over-consumed toxins. Everyone wonders why the "sick" waiting area at the pediatrician's office is full and overcrowded, while the media and pharmaceutical industry have us believe that it's "flu" season.

In order to avoid these kinds of episodes, we always pack and prepare our kids' lunches, to ensure proper food and nutrition. We ask the teachers to notify us in advance as much as possible of special occasions so we could send an alternative organic snack or treat with our kids so they could still partake in the activities and not feel left out. We also check our children's nerve system on a weekly basis to see if they need a chiropractic adjustment, to make sure their spine is in proper alignment so their nervous system is functioning at optimal levels. Our family's belief system? We believe that the healthy habits and sacrifices that we make today, though others may not choose them, will allow our family to have the health benefits that others unfortunately won't have in the future.

This is the part of the book where some might be tempted to put down the book and write us off as fanatics. What's so wrong with one cupcake or a slice of birthday cake? Honestly, not that much, but it's the cumulative effect of day after day, week after week, year after year that causes this generation of current children to have the highest rates of diabetes, obesity and sickness in history. It's the constant toxic overload of processed foods, fast foods, sugar, hormones, antibiotics, artificial sweeteners, artificial dyes and colorings in their food supply that ultimately causes early onset of so many chronic diseases. Did you know the average American eats fast food four to five times per week? That's over 200 meals per year at fast food restaurants, where they are getting their maximum intake of "junk."—the average fast food meal has 1200 calories! Have we gotten to the point where we are teaching our kids that eating out of a bag is acceptable and normal? Obesity is a huge problem facing our culture today. The CDC states that more than 30 percent of kids are overweight and studies have shown that when children eat fast food once a week, they gained about six pounds more per year than did their peers who did not eat fast food.

Families come in to us to get chiropractic adjustments and while getting the kids adjusted, we hear questions about mucus overload, allergies and unexplained symptoms and sickness. The medical answer is pharmaceuticals to cover up and suppress the symptoms and ultimately increase the toxic stress on the body. Our answer is to remove nerve interference through specific, scientific chiropractic adjustments, which we consider to be the most crucial aspect of keeping your babies and kids healthy and well. However if you keep feeding your baby or children "junk", their bodies will show signs of toxicity and immune distress.

We're not suggesting that you can never have fast food, as we all are on the run at times, but consider the amount of times you feed the kids this overly processed "food made by man." Is a once or twice a week stop at the local fast food joint too much? That's something you'll have to decide for yourself and your family, but we believe that most kids are overloaded and toxic with chemicals found in processed food, many of which come from fast food restaurants. Furthermore, some people seem to think that certain fast food places are "healthier" than others, holding a kind of "tiering" system for fast food, which makes it okay to take the kids through certain drive thrus—after all, they're getting a semi-nutritious meal, right? But junk food is junk food whether you like it or not and our advice for healthy babies and kids is to avoid it all as much as possible. Fast food should only be used in cases of emergency, like a flight delay at the airport where you're stuck without real food, or during a road trip in the middle of nowhere. Don't get us wrong, we've been in some pinches before where we had to sacrifice and feed the kids questionable food. That being said, when you're a few miles from the house and just in a hurry and ill-prepared, your baby and kids will pay with ill health. Preparation is as easy as bringing fruit and healthy snacks when you're going around town and making food in advance at home so you avoid getting into a fast food fix.

Another place to watch our children's food intake is at daycare or preschool. A parent might assume that the school is doing their best to provide nutritious food to our precious little ones. The truth is, they are, but in their warped opinion of good food and the current food pyramid. If a school administrator who monitors the program has bad food habits themselves, then they may honestly see nothing wrong with feeding the kids highly processed foods. Not to mention that the school has a budget and bulk amounts of high sugar, starchy, processed foods is always the cheaper way to feed a lot of people. We don't even own a microwave at our home, so we heat up our kids' food in the morning and place it in a thermos container to avoid the line at the microwave in the lunchroom. We attempted to purchase small ovens for the lunchroom as an alternative to the microwave, but we were told they would be a fire hazard and it is not allowed to bring in food to heat in the cafeteria kitchen ovens, as that would be against health department regulations.

The truth is that most people just don't know that there is a better way to eat and live and that's what the Designed by God cause is all about! We believe if people knew what we knew, then they would do what we do. When we visit the preschool and see them wheeling the cart of hormone and antibiotic-laden milk and sugar-filled cookies to the kids for their mid-morning snack, we just cringe. Parents don't realize how bad this food is when eaten on a continual basis. This gives us the passion to write this book and provide knowledge for parents who are looking for it. These children truly are perishing for their parent's lack of knowledge. Remember 1 Corinthians 6:19: "Do you not know that your bodies are temples of the Holy Spirit, who is in you, whom you have received from God? You are not your own."

Natural Birth:
The Road Less Traveled
by Charity Haulk and Dr. Amanda Hess.

One day in my sixth grade English class my teacher, Mr. Likins gave the class an assignment. We had to choose a poem from the poetry book, memorize it and recite it in front of the class the following week. I chose the poem, "The Road Not Taken," by Robert Frost. The poem is about a person who sees two roads in the woods, both equally traveled, but cannot decide what road to take. Both roads look the same and one would like to travel both. The person sighs with regret, that he or she may never have a chance to travel down that other road. At the end of the poem, the person takes the road less traveled by and it has made all the difference.

The same is true when choosing a birthing road. There are two roads: The Natural Birth Road and the Medicated Birth Road and every woman that becomes pregnant, chooses one of these roads. When I became pregnant with my first born, Ethan, I chose the Medicated road. This was the popular choice. Everyone I knew was induced with Pitocin and was given an epidural. My mom was the only person I knew who had natural births. She would tell me stories of how she had very little pain, only pressure after her water had broke. She easily and naturally gave birth to me, my sister and my brother. She encouraged me to have Ethan naturally, that it was the best for both of us. I remember telling her that I didn't want to feel anything.

94

Why would I want to have a potentially "painful" birth, when I could get an epidural and feel nothing. She would tell me that God has given pain and pressure, so I would be able to feel to push out the baby and every drug that I would receive, my baby would also get. I couldn't believe this was true. My midwife and doctor would never give me nor the baby something that could be potentially harmful or have long term effects. My husband and I trusted that they would only make decisions based on what was best for me and our baby.

The medical birth model believes that the drugs given during birth like an Epidural are localized to the spine, having no effect on the baby giving the mother control over her body and a break from labor. The natural birth model believes that all drugs given during labor affect the mother and the baby potentially causing short term and long term effects and should only be given in the event that a true life-threatening condition arises. The medicated road is portrayed as painless, harmless and easier for everyone. Having traveled both roads, I can tell you that the medicated birth road is not what it appears to be.

When my husband and I arrived at the hospital around 4:30 pm, we parked in the parking deck and walked across the breezeway to the hospital and took the elevator to the maternity wing of the hospital. When we checked in, the medical staff gave us some paper work to fill out.

One of the pages we had to fill out was called "Consent to Routine Procedures & Treatments". The consent form states, *"During the course of my care and treatment, I understand that various types of tests, diagnostic or treatment procedures ("Procedures") may be necessary. These Procedures may be performed by physicians, nurses, technologists, technicians, physician assistants or other healthcare professionals. The next paragraph goes on to state, "While routinely performed without incident, there may be material risks associated with each of these Procedures. I understand that it is not possible to list every risk or every Procedure and that this form only attempts to identify the most common material risks and the alternatives (if any) associated with the Procedures. I also understand that various Healthcare Professionals may have differing opinions as to what constitutes material risks and alternative Procedures".*

The form goes on to list the Procedures that may have to be performed, but are not limited to these five;

1. Needle Sticks
2. Physical tests, assessments and treatments
3. Administration of Medications
4. Drawing blood, Bodily fluids or Tissue Samples
5. Insertion of Internal Tubes

Under each Procedure was included the possible material risks associated with each one. The word "Material Risks" in laymen's terms means, "Physical/Bodily Risks". To most people the words "material risks" does not sound as scary as physical risks. The "material" they were talking about was my body that was carrying my precious little baby. The consent form never mentioned that any of these Procedures could possibly cause any "physical risks" to Ethan, my baby. The second page of the consent form stated, By signing this form:

I consent to Healthcare Professionals performing Procedures as they deem reasonably necessary or desirable in the exercise of their professional judgement, including those Procedures that may be unforeseen or not known to be needed at the time this consent is obtained; and

2. I acknowledge that I have been informed in general terms of the nature and purpose of the Procedure; the material risk of the Procedures; and practical alternatives to the Procedures.

3. If I have any questions or concerns regarding these Procedures, I will ask my physician to provide me with additional information. I also understand that my physician may ask me to sign additional informed Consent Documents.

Looking back I do not remember even reading what the consent form said. When you are at the hospital preparing to have a baby, you are not interested in reading or analyzing paper work. I just wanted to get checked in and settled into a room. I trusted that whatever medication or procedures that might be done to me was for my own good. That they would inform me of what they were going to do before they did it. Once we got to the room, I was asked to change out of all my clothes and put on a hospital gown. They then took my blood pressure and temperature. A young inexperienced nurse then tried to start my IV line on my left wrist, but after four failed attempts, had to call a more experienced nurse who came in and started one on my right wrist, after the first try. Late that night around midnight my midwife came into my room and told me that I needed to get some rest and that she would give "something to help me sleep". I said, "Ok, sounds great", I thought I could just sleep until my contractions started or my water broke. At that time I was never told what I would be given. I later found out that they had given me Ambien. After blindly taking the

Ambien, I had an allergic reaction to the drug that caused me four hours of itching, scratching, shaking, dizziness and hallucinations.

The next morning I got a new midwife... A woman I had never met before. She came in and broke my water. I then was given an epidural, followed by Pitocin through my IV. While I felt nothing because of the paralyzing and weakening effect the epidural had on my body—Ethan, however, was receiving seven times the dose recommended for his tiny 7 pound 14 oz body. For six straight hours he was being squeezed by the unnaturally strong contractions that Pitocin causes and suffocated over and over again from the high doses of continual administration of Pitocin. This is why so many babies end up in distress during a Pitocin induced labor.

When I finally dilated to 10 centimeters, they told me to start pushing. Since I couldn't feel any contractions, I artificially depended on the monitor, staff and my family to tell me when to push. I was laying almost flat on my back, with my feet up in the stirrups. The midwife mentioned that I may have to have a C-section, because I wasn't pushing well enough. I repeatedly told them I couldn't feel anything to push. But nobody listened to me. It was like I was invisible. They wouldn't turn off the Pitocin or even turn it down. They kept telling me to bear down like I was having a bowel movement. I tried pushing with all I had. But I was exhausted. It had been 24 hours since I was allowed to eat or drink anything. After three and a half hours of pushing, Ethan went into fetal distress. His heart tones were dropping. Then without my knowledge they screwed the vacuum extractor to his head and tried to pull him out. His head came out, but his shoulders got stuck, this is called shoulder dystocia. With Ethan's head hanging limp out of my body, the midwife struggled to free his shoulders. When she couldn't get him out, the nurse to the right of me "jumped" on top of my stomach, pushing down with her right knee, at the same time the midwife called a code pink and gave me a level 4 episiotomy, an incision where they cut from your perineum to your anus. When they finally got him out, he was not breathing.

Ethan was lifeless and white as a sheet. My grandmother who was also in the room thought he was still born. Asking my husband to step aside, the midwife carried his limp body over to a table. She and several other nurses immediately began to resuscitate him.

While they were saving my son, I laid there paralyzed, barely able to see over my feet, wondering what was happening. I could feel the tension in the air. I knew something was wrong when my husband and my mother started to cry. I could hear one of the nurses say, "breathe, buddy breathe." It was several minutes before they brought him back to life as he was gasping as he took his first breath.

Informed Consent

The definition of "consent" is permission for something to happen or agreement to do something.[1] The definition of "informed consent" is legal procedure to ensure that a patient, client and research participants are aware of all the potential risks and costs involved in a treatment or procedure. It informs the client of the nature of the treatment, possible alternative treatments and the potential risks and benefits of the treatment.[2]

---

[1] http://www.oxforddictionaries.com/us/definition/american_english/consent
[2] http://psychology.about.com/od/iindex/g/def_informedcon.htm

The AMA (American Medical Association) describes Informed Consent as more than simply getting a patient to sign a written consent form. It is a process of communication between a patient and physician and the information on the consent form should be disclosed and discussed by the physician and not a delegated representative like a hospital employee or nurse.

In turn, the patient should have an opportunity to ask questions to require a better understanding of the treatment or procedure, so that he or she can make an informed decision to proceed or to refuse a particular course of medical intervention.

The AMA goes on to describe informed consent as both an ethical obligation and a legal requirement spelled out in statutes and case law in all 50 states. The AMA's Code of Medical Ethics also states that physicians must provide relevant information to their patients. This information protects the patient. It gives them freedom to make their own choices about what is done to their body and how it is done.

Sadly. . . this does not happen in most healthcare facilities especially in the area of maternity care and childbirth. Parents are given very little information. Most of the time they do not realize the risk associated with the procedures and protocols within the facility. True Informed Consent lays everything out on the table. It ensures that the mother is aware of all the potential risks and side effects of all medications, treatments and procedures. In order for informed consent to be considered valid, the mother must be competent of the material she is signing and the consent should be given voluntarily.[3]

[3] http://legal-dictionary.thefreedictionary.com/Patients'+Rights

The Importance of Informed Consent

Although I did sign the consent form voluntarily, we did not fully understand or have complete knowledge of all the possible side effects or physical risks for myself or Ethan. We were never given any information during our prenatal office visits about the birthing process, the medications given, or routine hospital procedures. Whenever a person is given a prescription from a doctor they have to go to a pharmacy to have it filled. By law the pharmacist has to include information about the drug and all the possible side effects. They are also warning about who should and should not be taking this drug.

The same type of guidelines should apply to labor. All healthcare providers should be required to provide parents with information regarding all procedures or protocols related to delivery. This should be given at the beginning of their prenatal office visits and not the day of delivery. They should also provide a list of all medications routinely used and their possible side effects. This would give parents time to research, ask providers additional questions and make a birth plan or guidelines about what is important to them and what they want to avoid.

Most people are taught growing up to trust in their provider. That their "doctor knows best!" This mindset continues into adulthood and then parenthood. But as parents, God wants us to exercise wisdom in all areas. As parents we have to be prepared and educated in every area of our lives, taking responsibility for our family's health.

I believe the road of natural birth is less traveled today because of the lack of true informed consent. Sadly parents are not fully informed by their provider of the risks of routine procedures or protocols performed during labor and delivery, nor the interventions that are caused because of them. They are not encouraged to take responsibility of their bodies and birth. Even taking a childbirth class and depending on the instructor and who is paying them may not even prepare a woman for birth. Lack of informed consent puts the provider in complete control. Because parents are not equipped with the truth, they are too fearful to question any drug given or procedure performed.

During Ethan's birth, I was never informed that anything was wrong. I had no idea that he was stuck or in distress. I never was told they were going to have to screw a vacuum extractor to his head to pull him out along with an episiotomy that would require over thirty stitches to sew up. No one asked my permission to do anything. Was this God's plan for me for my birth? NO! Looking back now after the fact, I don't believe it was. That is why informed consent is so important. I would have never chosen to give my son all those drugs if I was fully informed of their ingredients and possible side effects. Should I have honored my mother and listened to her Godly and biblical advice about birth and labor? YES! I believe things would have gone differently for me during his birth. Some of you reading this book may have a mom or a close friend or family member speaking these same truths of God's Natural Birth Plan into your life. Listen to them! Be proactive about your birth. Interview providers, find one that believes in natural birth. Pick a birthplace where you feel the most comfortable, a place that will respect your wishes about childbirth and work with you to make your birth a joyful experience. Take childbirth education classes that will educate you and give you tools that will help prepare you for birth. Most importantly surround yourself with people who believe in the power of natural birth.

As soon as we left the hospital with Ethan, we drove to Drs. Hess' office before going home so he could get his first specific chiropractic adjustment. We knew his neck was for sure out of alignment after the vacuum suction, hematoma on his skull from the suction and shoulder dystocia.

Ethan was born in August 2006. A few months later in April 2007, Dr. Amanda Hess had given birth to Alyssa, her first born. I distinctly remember coming to the office for our regular chiropractic check up for myself and Ethan, when a conversation happened that forever changed my life. I asked Dr. Amanda how her birth went, expecting a similar story as mine. But that wasn't the case at all. She looked at me with a sparkle in her eyes and a smile that lit up the room. She gave birth to Alyssa at her house with no medications, no interventions and no tearing. She was sore, but she felt on top of the world. Immediately I wanted to cry. I thought about how I missed out and about how that was the kind of birth that I had wanted not only for myself but also for my baby. Outside of my mother, Dr. Amanda was the only other person I knew that had chosen this path.

For the births of our next two children, we chose a different path.... the road less traveled by... natural birth. Both of our children, Lauren and Hayden, were born at home with no interventions necessary. I felt every contraction and my body told me when it was time to push. Both labors were faster than my artificial medicated labor with Ethan and both labors were uncomplicated. Unlike the person in the Robert frost poem,I do not look back on our decision to go a different road. I do not wonder if we made the right choice. Choosing to birth naturally has made all the difference in our lives and the lives of our children. On this new road I learned about the way God made and designed a woman, the truth about our bodies and birth and the how God has given parents the responsibility and authority over their children's lives. Through His word, he has equipped us with the knowledge to make the best decisions for our family.

5.
Chemical Soup

When walking into a grocery store, many labels on food claim one product to be better for us than another product and lots of marketing and media has confused the public on what's really worth the extra expense and effort. Organic foods are a prime example of this, so let's jump in and explore them. If a food or product has a label calling it organic, this implies that it is grown, or its ingredients are grown or made, without the use of pesticides or chemical fertilizers. It also means that the item is not processed using irradiation, industrial solvents, or chemical food additives. Now, sometimes a product might claim to be "made with organic ingredients," which typically means that 70 percent or more of its ingredients are organic and the ingredients label will tell you which are and which are not. The organic industry is a very regulated industry and a certified USDA Organic label is what you need to look for to be certain of the product's claims. You might also look for words like "hormone free", "antibiotic free", "preservative free", "non GMO" and "chemical free".

Why invest the extra money to buy organic? For starters, it is widely known among scientists and researchers that the chemicals used in commercial agriculture practices for non-organic food cause cancer! Some think that "organic" is hype, but research consistently shows increased rates of all types of cancer and immune diseases linked to pesticides, herbicides, fungicides, insecticides and synthetic chemicals. Non-organic producers use these substances to increase crops and agriculture production of foods and animals.[1] Are you aware that 60 percent of all herbicides are carcinogenic (cancer causing), 90 percent of all fungicides are carcinogenic and 30 percent of all pesticides are carcinogenic? Non-organic dairy, poultry and meats use a variety of hormones and antibiotics, which harm the body, cause many endocrine diseases and weaken and destroy our immune system. It's no wonder so many of our babies and kids are sick, symptomatic and suffering, due to parents not realizing the short- and long-term harm they are causing their babies, toddlers and children by consuming this harsh and invasive "chemical soup."

Unknown to many parents as well, non-organic food typically goes through "irradiation," which means that ionizing radiation is used to kill certain microorganisms. However, with irradiation, some nutrients in the food can be destroyed and by-products like "unique radiolytic products" can be created in the foods, which in many cases increases the toxicity of the food. Some of these by-products are chemicals that have yet to be identified. Yuck! The last thing anybody wants is for their fruits and vegtables to be essentially "microwaved" or irradiated. The

[1] http://www.shapefit.com/diet/10-reasons-eat-organic.html

way we want to eat our food is like it was in the Garden of Eden, or close to that as presently possible, pure and unsullied at the source.

The choice is yours. It does force you to prepare and make your own food, which clearly isn't such a bad idea. Choosing to feed your family organic foods is a great health decision because you avoid all types of chemicals, antibiotics, hormones and toxins. Children seem to be more vulnerable to these chemicals and the long term consequences of consuming non-organic foods is yet to be determined, but with the trends of cancer, autoimmune diseases and common childhood conditions on the rise, we believe these toxic substances found in processed, non-organic, or fast food are on the top of the list as a causative factor. A positive side effect of your family's choice to go organic as much as possible is an effect on the air, water and soil quality, as organic farming has very little negative effect compared to all the chemical spill-off and contamination of non-organic farming. Also, much of organic farming is being done by local, smaller and non-commercial farmers, so buying organic typically supports small farmers.

Toxins Lurking around the House

Our homes are full of toxins, many of which are impossible to avoid, but we're going to take a closer look at the ones we think are avoidable and have the most negative effect on our babies and children. Some of these toxins we review are quite familiar around our homes and our families have been using them for years. At first mention of them, you might be startled like we were when we started our research about fifteen or so years ago.

We had a hard time believing that the products our family had used for as long as we could remember were actually dangerous and needed to be avoided. Our advice as we go through this part of "Chemical Soup", is to keep an open mind and then follow up with your own research and you too just might be making the switch to non-toxic and chemical free.

We all know that no one has more sensitive and fragile skin as a newborn baby, yet did you realize that dozens of popular baby shampoos and skincare products have some lethal chemicals in them? Two of the most concerning chemicals are formaldehyde and 1,4 dioxane.[2] Formaldehyde is considered a known carcinogen by government scientists and 1,4 dioxane has been shown to cause cancer in animal studies. If you're using common bath products from your local drug or grocery store, you can bet you're lathering up your kids with these toxins everyday. An amazing and easy-to-use online source for knowing what's in all your skin and hair care products is EWG. org. The Environmental Working Group is the nation's leading environmental health research and advocacy organization. EWG is a non-profit and researches many consumable products, including the foods we eat, the water we drink and the skincare products we put on our bodies. Their website will open your eyes to the chemicals and toxins used or not used in the products we use on our children and ourselves. Their "Cosmetic Database" lists the chemicals in each product and rates products by their toxicity. The best part of the EWG website is that not only can you see what *not* to buy, but their research also shows you which products are the safest, giving you a practical solution and products to purchase and use.

---

[2] http://www.nytimes.com/2012/08/16/business/johnson-johnson-to-remove-formaldehyde-from-products.html?_r=0

EWG and many other researchers have also pointed to sunscreen as another product that is loaded with carcinogenic and harmful chemicals. Sunscreen is seriously toxic and all parents should carefully research and choose a safe sunscreen. Retinyl palmitate is one chemical found in 25 percent of all beach and sport sunscreens. It is thought to be photocarcinogenic, so when it is lathered on the skin and then exposed to the sun, it speeds the growth of skin tumors. We're not kidding here—25 percent of sunscreens actually accelerate the development of skin tumors and lesions on sun exposed skin![3] Oxybenzone, another toxic industrial chemical found in nearly half of sunscreens, is potentially disruptive to our hormones and triggers allergic skin reactions in sensitive individuals. While sunscreens are certainly necessary, just make sure you are using the safest ones possible on your children and yourself. Go to EWG.org to make the best choice for you and your family.

Now it is time for everyone to take a deep breath. This is difficult terrain for most of us parents, as we start realizing the damage being currently done to our children. The good news is you can do something about this today by changing the habits you have and the products you buy. You can become informed and help other families get informed as well. We wrote this book so that all of God's children are informed and have a choice, as you start to understand that there is a better way.

Unfortunately, we must continue our exploration of the toxins you may be using. This next topic will be tough to swallow, since it's been very ingrained into our heads how good it is supposed to be for us. The culprit? Fluoride. How could

[3] http://expatdoctormom.com/2011/06/dangers-of-sunscreen/

fluoride possibly be harmful to us when the American Dental Association (ADA), our favorite dentist, our favorite toothpaste company and even our elementary school nurse has been telling us for as long as we can remember that fluoride is the best thing for our teeth? It's even supposed to be beneficial in our water.[4] However, hundreds of research projects done on fluoride have revealed its dangers, which include male reproductive system damage, lowered IQ, fetal brain damage, behavioral issues, bone damage, increased incidence of hip fractures in the elderly, thyroid dysfunction, bone cancer in young males and even the early onset of puberty in children. Its toxicity rates in babies have gotten so bad that even the ADA released an email in 2006 to its members warning that in order to prevent tooth damage, flouridated water should not be mixed into formula or foods intended for babies aged 1 and younger.[5] "Infants could receive a greater than optimal amount of fluoride through liquid concentrate or powdered baby formula that has been mixed with water containing fluoride during a time that their developing teeth may be susceptible to enamel fluorosis," describing the condition marked by pitting and white spotting as well as yellow and/or brown teeth."[6] In fact, most developed countries, including Japan and the majority of western Europe, do not consume fluoridated water.

And yet, even with all this research showing the detrimental effects of fluoride, the American food supply is inundated with the substance. It's in our water, juice, soda, wine and coffee, in soups and processed food and in toothpastes and baby formula.

[4] http://www.cheeseslave.com/top-10-dangers-of-fluoride/

[5] http://www.naturalnews.com021072_fluoridated_water_fluoride.html#ixzz2hVgcFNYN

[6] http://www.naturalnews.com021072_fluoridated_water_fluoride.html#ixzz2hVbEWiA9.

Most American cities also have fluoridated water. The first thing to do is to buy fluoride-free toothpaste and fluoride-free products when you can and invest in a water filter that removes fluoride from your water supply. Check out the Flouride Action Network's website, flourideAlert.org, to help guide and direct you through this well-known chemical with unknown toxicity.

Everyone has seen the sign: "Wash your hands before you go back to work." Now that's good advice and we always wonder if (and hope that) the employees at those food establishments actually do. Washing hands with soap and water is one of those things you train your kids to do, like brushing their teeth or how to tie their shoes. However, in this germaphobic society we live in, things have gotten a bit out of control with "killing germs." The newest invention now carried in all diaper bags and purses—and displayed in every classroom in America—is hand sanitizer. As most of us know, germs (microorganisms, bacteria, fungi and so forth) serve a purpose and that's why God created them. So what's the deal with germs and why all the hoopla? The truth is, if the germ theory of disease were true, none of us would be here talking about it. Look at it this way: Germs are everywhere, but they thrive in dirty or poorly taken care of environments. For example, if you had a garbage dump a quarter mile down the street from your home, where would you find more flies, at the dump or in your home? The obvious answer is at the garbage dump, because it's dirty, whereas your home is a much cleaner environment. The same is true with germs. They are everywhere, but they only thrive and manifest in a junkyard environment, or in a body where the immune system is suppressed and when the body is not properly taken care of.

So, if we do things like have proper food intake and nutrition, get routine specific chiropractic care, exercise and maintain health-conscious habits, then our immune systems will have a much higher resistance and our bodies will function the way God intended them to. Why is it that one person can have a cold and sleep in the same bed as another person, but that other person never catches the cold virus? Because the other person's immune system was not compromised and therefore, the cold virus could not thrive in that person's body.

However, since the media has created germaphobia among so many people, we now have dangerous chemicals being used by us and our children many times a day. They're called "antibacterial" soaps and hand sanitizers.[7] ABC News recently reported that scientists are questioning the use of antibacterial products and specifically the chemicals in the products themselves, as almost 50 percent of all soaps on the market have antibacterial agents in them. Chemicals called triclosan and triclocarban, which are used in these type of products (though they have never had any published research that it is more effective than soap and water), have been shown to kill good bacteria that the body needs. Not only that, but research is showing that these chemicals can cause "super bugs" and create an environment where these mutated bacteria are more likely to survive. Triclosan and triclocarban are linked to endocrine dysfunction, brain damage and several types of cancer.[8] Triclosan has never received a formal safety approval from the FDA and it is not only found in hand sanitizers and soaps, but toothpastes, children's toys and many other consumer products.

[7] http://abcnews.go.com/Health/story?id=117985&page=1#.UZGsrL_BqfQ

[8] http://www.naturalnews.com/040298_triclosan_antibacterial_soaps_FDA_review.html

We tell our children not to use the antibacterial hand sanitizer at school or anywhere and that just warm water and normal soap is fine. Scientists and researchers have been saying this all along and the push to promote antibacterial hand sanitizer is just another marketing ploy to sell products. Think about how many places you see those hand sanitizers hanging on the walls of our churches, schools, airports, day cares and baby nurseries, just to name a few. Well-meaning parents smear this stuff all over their babies and kids, not knowing that it is another toxic, cancer-causing chemical that can be easily avoided. It's just so sad to see all these products used so frequently and everyone thinks they are doing the right thing.

We spent a long weekend at Disney World recently and all we could see was these parents unknowingly smearing gobs of sunscreen and hand sanitizer on their babies and children, never suspecting that these are very carcinogenic chemicals. All we could imagine is many of them saying to us, "Why has no one ever told us that continued use of these products can be harmful to our children?"

One chemical that you may have heard of, one which is widely found in plastic products that are exposed to our children, is Bisphenol A or BPA. If you look closely at plastic products like baby bottles or plastic containers, you might have seen some of the companies advertise "BPA free". Typically, plastic items containing BPA are marked with a 7 on the bottom for recycling purposes. As a guide, plastics marked with a 1, 2, 4, or 5 on the bottom are classified as safe, while plastics with 3, 6, or 7 are not safe and should be avoided. A good rule of thumb is to use plastic as little as possible. When we are at home, in the car, or at the chiropractic office, we drink our water from glass containers. If we're traveling, we try to buy water that's contained in glass. When we cook or prepare food at the house and store it in the refrigerator or take it to work, we always use glass or porcelain and our kids' water is in stainless steel when they go to school.[9] The Mayo Clinic reports that plastic products containing BPA should be used cautiously and that alternatives such as glass, porcelain or stainless steel are much better options. They also warn consumers to never microwave or heat food in plastics, as the chemicals can leach into food. BPA has been linked to brain, behavioral and prostate gland issues in fetuses, infants and children. Recent studies show this current generation of children are testing with high amounts of BPA in their urine. These studies also suggest that this could be linked to kidney disease, heart disease and obesity in children.

How much do you pay for water? If you're like us, you're spending way too much. Studies approximate that the average American buys 167 bottles of water every year, spending about $250 a year. At your home, we recommend a home water filtration system that filters all the water in your house—or at minimum, buy an under-the-sink reverse osmosis system to use in the kitchen. When you're buying water for you and the kids to drink, look at the label. Don't buy store brands labeled as "purified water". These types of water are safe to drink, it's just that they are actually tap water that is taken from a public water main, put through a reverse osmosis process and marketed as "pure water." If you have to buy water, purchase some that is from an actual natural spring source. Examine the label to see what the source of the water is. We recommend for many reasons that spring water is better for you and the kids.

You might be getting overloaded at this point. There are some other hot topics that we want you to be aware of, like harsh chemicals found in cleaning products, the drawbacks of milk, how to properly read food labels and some other extremely helpful guidance and tips. We've created a *Baby Designed by God* resource section in the back of the book to help you weed through these and many other topics and areas of concern.

Some people will argue the small amount of these chemicals present in products is no cause for you to worry, but we see the long-term, cumulative effect of these toxins as the issue. Small amounts of toxins from multiple sources add up, whether in toxic foods, plastics, cleaning products, vaccines, pharmaceuticals, skin care and the like. They all add up to an amount that causes many babies and toddlers to reach toxic levels and present physical illness and ailments. These in turn are treated with more toxic pharmaceuticals! Yes, you have to pick your battles and we all must do our best to eliminate chemical exposure to our children as much as possible. It does take time to learn what's best for our babies and children, to prepare the best foods and avoid toxins and to choose the best care, but aren't your children worth the extra effort and sacrifice? We believe that our children were designed by God and given to us by Him and it's our responsibility to "start children off on the way they should go, and even when they are old they will not turn from it." Proverbs 22:6 (NIV)

Lincoln's Birth Story
By Dana Brower

I had the best pregnancy. From the moment I found out I was pregnant until my 38-week checkup with my midwife, everything was perfect. My husband and I decided very early on in our pregnancy to plan for an at-home waterbirth with the assistance of a midwife and doula. This plan was in place up until my due date and the last visit I had with my midwife.

At my 38-week checkup, my midwife did her normal "testing." She took my urine sample with a urine stick, measured my belly, listened to the baby, weighed me and took my blood pressure. My blood pressure was 130/84, but the week prior it had been 112/80. This started a whole bunch of blood work and urine testing that I had never planned on. I was informed at this time (correctly or incorrectly) that I was developing preeclampsia. I felt perfectly fine, with no symptoms of preeclampsia whatsoever (characterized by high blood pressure and significant amounts of protein in the urine of a pregnant woman, usually associated with swelling of hands, face and feet), just the higher blood pressure. The midwife advised us that we would now need to come in for a visit every two to three days. My blood pressure continued to rise at each visit and it was in the 130s over 90 each time we took it; however, I never had protein in my urine or any other "symptoms" of preeclampsia.

The night going into my due date, I had regular contractions every five to seven minutes. I ended up spending the night awake in the bathtub extremely uncomfortable and just feeling "off." I finally woke up my husband at about 7 am and explained the discomfort. He expressed that I should relax and try to nap before we visited the midwife at noon.

As we left for this visit, a light snow had started to fall and the forecasters were calling for a blizzard that evening. This midwife visit would be the most stressful moment of my entire pregnancy. After taking my blood pressure, which was 132/90 and measuring my belly, the midwife decided she would no longer attend a homebirth and I needed to be induced in a hospital. My husband was less then thrilled. He had strongly supported my desire to have a homebirth and avoid medical intervention. We both wanted to do this naturally in a comfortable environment.

This decision made by my midwife left me very tense and shaken about what to do next. When everyone finally took a moment to calm down, I decided that we should just go to a hospital birthing center and proceed from there. Thankfully, our midwife did have acquaintances who were midwives at both of the hospitals in the area that have birthing centers.

She was able to call over and see which hospital had doctors and teams that were "friendly" toward couples who had been planning homebirths. Though we didn't realize it at the time, her decision and discretion was one of the biggest blessings we would receive in regards to labor. The hospital that had been our first choice for in case of emergency transfer due to location and atmosphere had a doctor on staff who was opposed to homebirth. The other hospital (a bit farther away) had a team that was comfortable with transfers, so we decided to go there.

By the time we left the midwife's office to head home to pack for a birth plan we never had planned for, it was snowing hard. When we finally were able to get on the road to head down to the hospital, it was a near white out. New York was officially in a blizzard. The 40-minute drive took an hour and a half.

We were able to go straight to labor and delivery and I was checked in right away and examined. My blood pressure was still the same and I now was going to meet the OB who would be taking over my care. I liked her: she understood that this was not what we wanted whatsoever, but it was no longer in our hands; we had to make the best decision for the baby and that meant he needed to come out.

She did an exam and I was two centimeters dilated and 80 percent effaced. This was extremely good news since we were now forced with induction. We had been educated that induction done at this stage is much less lengthy and more likely to work than when done at one centimeter or less. I still did not see this as a reason to celebrate; however, at that point I was concerned with avoiding as many interventions as possible, especially a C-section. I was asked about pain medication and I told the doctor that in no way did I want anything. She basically told me I had no idea what I was getting myself into with a Pitocin induction and the pain levels that it would cause. In pregnancy circles, Pitocin is also known as liquid hell.

Now, this is where I must say that we were truly blessed with our midwife's choice for this hospital and doctor. The doctor wanted to know what we wished for in our birth plan. For me, I wanted to labor in the bathtub in the room and be able to move around and not be confined to the hospital bed. My husband wanted to delay cutting the cord so the placental blood could all be transferred to our newborn to avoid anemia at birth and provide higher iron levels during infancy. He also told the doctor to not pull the baby's head and neck out forcefully like we had seen in so many pictures and videos. Thankfully, our doctor agreed to all of the above.

Our homebirth midwife arrived right after they started the Pitocin IV. It was just about 5 pm. She was shocked to find out I was getting ready to get in the tub. It is unheard of to allow someone on Pitocin to go off of constant fetal monitoring; however, our baby was not having any dips in heart rate, so we were allowed to move. I believe most women have no idea that this is even an option. I labored in the tub for the next three hours. When I was checked at this point, I was only three centimeters dilated, I was in immense pain and the contractions were almost constant due to the Pitocin. It felt that each Pitocin contraction worked into the next. The decision then was made to break my water (I was not asked if I wanted this or not). If I thought I was in pain before, this was a nightmare. The contractions became ten times worse, if that was even possible.

I had reached a threshold where I really was considering pain medication. Again, though, another blessing occurred. I was informed I could not get any pain medications due to the results of my lab work. I had an extremely low platelet count, which ruled out an epidural. So, I just tried to survive each contraction. I was in so much pain, everything became a blur. A few hours later I experienced a change in pain and vomited several times. Shortly after the vomiting, I experienced an urge to push.

It was 11:40 pm when I started to push. I made the conscious decision not to listen to anyone in the room (it was a blizzard outside, so literally the staff was snowed in at the hospital, leading to a room full of nurses). I just listened to my body. I pushed when I felt I should and rested when my body told me to stop. At 12:01 am, Lincoln was born. I was able to hold our son on my chest and start to nurse him while we waited for the placenta to be delivered. My husband did not cut the cord until after the placenta was delivered and the pediatrician did not check the baby until after the cord was cut and I was finished nursing. The best part was that my husband never left my or our son's side. Lincoln then received his first chiropractic check up and adjustment, to make sure his nervous system was functioning at optimal levels. And our baby is perfect!

6.
Mother's Milk:
God's Free Gift

Have you ever wondered if the food you eat is made by God? Or, is it just man made? What's the difference and does it really matter? We believe food matters. Not only does food matter, but the source of your food matters. The substances and processes that are used to make your food also matter. You and your baby depend on it! Growth and function both rely on proper food and nutrition. What ramifications does the food you eat during pregnancy or nursing have on your baby? Do you really know what you are feeding your baby?

Due to the marketing agenda of the many food manufacturers, the food supply available has gotten very confusing and in some cases, completely out of hand. For example, virtually all of us reading this book would agree that we want to limit antibiotic use for our babies and ourselves. However, as reported by the John Hopkins School of Public Health, 80 percent of the antibiotics sold in the United States are sold for use in animal agriculture[1], meaning they are fed to animals, usually not to fight infection,

---

[1] http://www.jhsph.edu/research/centers-and-institutes/johns-hopkins-center-for-a-livable-future/about/focus_areas/antibiotic_res.html

but to make them bulk up more quickly. These antibiotics in the animal's feed remain in the animal and, after slaughter, they end up in our food supply and thus in ourselves and our babies. So many antibiotics are being used now, whether it's the 80 percent in the food supply or the 20 percent prescribed by doctors, that the CDC has recently declared the emerging antibiotic resistance issue a "nightmare." The Chief Medical Officer of the UK said in her 2011 annual report that antibiotic resistance is a "catastrophic threat" that poses a national security risk as serious as terrorism.[2]

Simply put, our food supply is seriously being tampered with. We are led to believe that the FDA and the U.S. government really have our best interests at heart, but this couldn't be further from the truth. The food supply maze that eventually leads to our babies and ourselves is long, confusing and disturbing, but let's take a closer look. There are a multitude of things to look at with our food supply. We can't cover all of these topics in one chapter, but we'll do our best to highlight some of the hot topics regarding food. There is recommended further reading on these topics in the Resource Guide at the back of the book.

God's First Food for Baby

First thing first: the best nutrition your baby will ever receive is its mother's breast milk. The good news is that the percentage of breastfeeding mothers has recently been increasing. Approximately 74.6 percent of women breastfeed their infant for any amount of time, with 44.4 percent breastfeeding for up to 6 months and 23.4 percent breastfeeding for up to 12

---

[2] http://www.wired.com/wiredscience/2013/03/uk-cmo-report/

months. Although breastfeeding is recommended for the first 12 months of life, the dramatic decline in these percentages as the infant gets older indicates that women need a better support system to allow them to breastfeed. From personal experience, I know it can be difficult and even stressful at times attempting to breastfeed your baby. Although I was fortunate to have both Alyssa and Gabriel with me at our practice everyday, it never seemed convenient or the "right time" to hear them crying and searching for the comfort and nourishment that only I could provide for them. I never fed my babies on a "schedule" or purposely let them cry it out. I always breastfed on demand, whether it was during the day or in the middle of the night. I have talked to many mothers who prefer different methods of breastfeeding. I just always say that the most important thing is that you are breastfeeding and not necessarily the method you use.

Breastfeeding my children, however, was an experience I will never forget. This divine yet helpless being that God gave me to take care of and raise up totally depended on me for nutrition, comfort and livelihood. After breastfeeding both my children for more or less the first two years of their lives, I am always thankful for that bonding time. Although there were many times I wanted to quit after being completely exhausted, my motherly love for my beloved children was the only thing that kept me going. I understand that there are valid reasons for not breastfeeding, such as adoption, orphaned babies, babies born to mothers with serious health problems, or a problem with the development of the mother's milk supply; however, I feel like moms who have the ability to breastfeed and just choose not to lose out for themselves and their baby.

There was one memorable evening that even I had to send my friend to the store for formula. I had eaten some chicken earlier that day and it didn't agree with me and by that evening I was doubled over the toilet vomiting with my stomach cramping. I felt dizzy and extremely weak. Then, I heard the cry of my constantly hungry son, Gabriel. I didn't even have the strength to hold him. I realized that I had used up all my freezer-stored breast milk, so my dear friend, Dr. Michael Viscarelli, attempted to save the day and ran to the store for me. He came back with Earth's Best infant formula and made a bottle for Gabriel. At the time, Gabriel was about 6 months old. Since birth, he had never tasted formula and only knew the taste and comfort of my milk. Dr. Michael did his best to try to satisfy Gabriel, as Jeremy was still at the office finishing up the day, but Gabriel was smarter than we realized. Gabriel knew we were trying to feed him the fake stuff. He spit it out at Dr. Michael's face, turned his mouth from the bottle and proceeded to scream at the top of his lungs in desperation for his mama. That night, Gabriel did cry himself to sleep while I rested with a glass of water next to me. A couple hours later, Gabriel woke up for his typical late night snack. By that time, I had recovered enough to breastfeed him back to sleep and all was well with mom and baby.

Now, making time for breastfeeding was a challenge during the day, with my busy schedule of adjusting practice members and handling the daily agenda at the practice. Like so many mothers, there were times of frustration and stress, when I knew my baby absolutely needed me, but other situations would crop up and try to pull me away from what I knew was necessary. I held my ground and fought for time to be with my baby, even when it meant saying a temporary no to other important people in my daily schedule. There were times when I knew I needed to plan ahead, like if I was going to speak about health principles at a church or business event, or had a meeting I couldn't miss. In those cases, I would schedule time during the day or at night to pump and store my milk in the freezer. Breast milk has a shelf life of about six months in the freezer, 72 hours in the refrigerator and four hours at room temperature, so I was sure to put my "liquid gold" in the freezer and store it for occasions when I either got desperate or knew I would be occupied and my baby needed some milk.

Women have a unique role of being a comforter to their children that men will never have the pleasure to experience. Although my mother was my comforter and I always searched for her and loved being with her, I know that my mother did not breastfeed me. I was a pure formula baby, with my mother believing her doctor 100 percent that formula was just as good and even better and more nutritious, than her own milk would be. My mother comes from the Baby Boomer generation, where many never question their doctor and instead do exactly what they say. I don't know if my mother regrets this aspect of mothering, but what I do know is that if she had been educated of the ingredients and inferior nutritional value of commercial formula, then maybe she would have made a different decision for my health. If a mother chooses not to breastfeed or cannot breastfeed for whatever reason, then she should seriously research the various homemade formula recipes available on websites, or books we recommend in the Resource Guide, which would be a far better solution with less toxic chemicals given to the baby.

Have you looked at the ingredients of most formulas lately? Virtually all brands of infant formulas, including "organic" and "natural" formulas, are loaded with corn syrup, sugar and a variety of oils.[3] They definitely do not contain the kind of stuff you want to give your baby. Most show the first ingredient as over 50 percent corn syrup solids, also know as high fructose corn syrup. This is almost like feeding your baby a can of soda. There are also reports of all sorts of questionable chemicals in infant formula. Chemicals like percholoric acid—the same chemical found in rocket fuel used in the defense and pyrotechnics industries—is found in formula. Bisphenol A (BPA), which has been linked to brain disorders, obesity and diabetes and could even be a factor in schizophrenia, is found in formula and many of our plastic products. Melamine, a white powder in some formulas that looks like powdered milk, has been linked to acute kidney failure; chronic exposure may cause cancer or reproductive damage. Soy-based formulas also pose a variety of health risks and 90 percent of soy is now genetically modified. Many studies show soy is linked to malnutrition, digestive distress, immune system breakdown, thyroid dysfunction, cognitive decline, reproductive disorders and infertility, cancer and heart disease. In fact, infants fed soy formula ingest an estimated five birth control pills' worth of estrogen every day.[4] Plus, many government agencies have ties to formula companies to promote formula, rather than breastfeeding, to lower-income mothers. In our fast-paced, fast food culture, formula is a temptation even for the most well

[3] http://www.naturalnews.com/033926_infant_formula_corn_syrup.html

[4] http://www.huffingtonpost.com/dr-mercola/soy-health_b_1822466.html

prepared mothers. Everyone wants what's best for her newborn and in this case, what is best is not what is expedient, but what God already designed us to do. If you look at the ingredients list on a can of formula and you cannot pronounce the words, you may want to think twice before feeding this to your baby on a daily basis.

Breast milk is the best food designed for baby and research shows that babies that are breast-fed for six months or more have better development, fewer illnesses and increased IQ. Research indicates children breast-fed longer than six months scored a 3.8-point IQ margin over those who were bottle-fed.[5] They also had increased immune function, which translates to less infections and less problems with allergies and has even been shown to protect against asthma and childhood cancers. Let's not forget one of the most important benefits of breastfeeding is the emotional bonding that happens with skin-to-skin contact between mom and baby.

Moms have lots of benefit from breastfeeding, too. For example, breastfeeding your baby increases the rate of weight loss, protects against early return of your menstrual cycle and presents less risk of immediate pregnancy with your next child. Breastfeeding increases levels of oxytocin, which stimulates postpartum uterine contractions and minimizes loss of blood flow.[6] I gained an average of 40 pounds with my pregnancies and breastfeeding not only allowed me to bond with each of my children, but also took off the pounds week by week. I am naturally a thin woman, but what I thought was crazy was that after having my children and breastfeeding for two years,

[5] http://www.scientificamerican.com/article.cfm?id=surety-bond-breast-feeding
[6] http://www.medelabreastfeedingus.com/benefits-of-breastfeeding

I weighed about five to eight pounds less than before I was pregnant. My menstrual cycle also did not return until both my children were each at 12 months of age. And the best thing about breastfeeding is that it costs nothing. It's a free gift from God. What a blessing—I get to lose weight, bond with my baby, prolong the return of my menstrual cycle and it's free!

AvaKate Birth Story
By Katie Guida

During lunchtime on the Friday before I gave birth, I began to have what I thought were Braxton-Hicks contractions (because of multiple false alarms). The contractions continued throughout the day, but they weren't that bad and I was not experiencing tightening in my abdomen, so I did not think that they were real contractions. This continued throughout the evening. I carried on about my night, making dinner, vacuuming the house, etc., only pausing when the contractions would hit. Around 11:30 pm while in the shower (to ease the gradually increasing pain), I began to have hot flashes.

At this point I realized that I was in transition, so I had my husband call the midwife, who was an hour away. She said she thought I was in labor but at that point wasn't sure how far along I was, so she began the trip down to our house. Around 12:45 am, I had an overwhelming urge to push. The closest place to give birth at that point was the bed, so I fell on my back and began to push.

After five pushes, I gave birth to a baby girl, with only my husband and mother in attendance. At 1:14 am, AvaKate was born healthy and loud, weighing 5 pounds 10 ounces. I look back now and think what an amazing testimony to specific chiropractic care my birth was, as I've been under chiropractic care since I was 13 years old due to migraines I once suffered from. Thankfully, my parents understood the benefits of having the whole family under chiropractic care as my siblings and I were growing up and I also received ongoing care throughout my pregnancy. I know that had much to do with my quick and fairly smooth birth.

My midwife arrived three minutes after my baby was born. For two hours, we were at home enjoying our new baby girl and then the midwife started to perform the newborn exam on my baby. She found a strange rhythm when listening to her heart and requested that we take her to the pediatrician to make sure that everything was okay. Well, being 3:00 in the morning, there was no pediatrician's office open, so our only other option was to take her to the ER. We took her to the local hospital in Henry County, Georgia and when we got there the nurses and hospital administration led us from the ER to the OBGYN floor and back down to the ER.

They didn't know what to do with us. This was about 45 minutes of walking, which wasn't easy considering I had just given birth. By the time they decided to send us back to the ER and we were registered, my baby's heart rate was very low because she was extremely cold. The ER doctor came in, performed routine tests, didn't explain much and told us to leave the room.

The nurse said that we did not want to stay in the room because it would be too difficult and we left feeling like we had no control. Once coming out of the room I was in tears, unsure of what was happening, so I sent my husband and father back in the room to find out. The ER doctor had decided to perform a tracheal intubation on my child, where they put a tube down the trachea to open up the airway. Once the procedure was complete, we were let back in the room. The ER doctor then proceeded to run more tests and then all of a sudden, the room was full of doctors and nurses who were in a panic because they said that my child did not have a blood pressure and yet she was obviously breathing.

The hospital made several mistakes during the time we were there with our newborn. The first mistake: They were checking her blood pressure with an adult machine, so it was not getting a proper reading on a small newborn. At this point, my child's breathing continued to become more and more abnormal, so we were told that they were going to have to transport her to another hospital that specialized in neonates. She was then transported to Emory Hospital in Midtown Atlanta.

At Emory Midtown, the on-call doctor did her best to get AvaKate stabilized. When looking at the paperwork from the emergency room, the doctor found that they had given my baby three times the dose of a sedative (needed for the intubation) as required for a newborn—this was their second mistake and what caused my baby's breathing to become sporadic. The doctor continued to work with my child to get her stabilized. She did not leave her side for eight hours until the sedative was out of her system. Sometime between 4 and 5 pm, there was a panic (which I was not made aware of until after) that my child stopped breathing for close to a minute.

By Sunday morning, my little baby was beginning to look like the child, rather than the supposed medical "disaster" that I gave birth to. She spent the next week in the NICU because she had to relearn how to latch on to my breast, because the intubation had numbed her senses and made it painful to swallow. Prior to the hospital visit, she had already latched on and breastfed within an hour of being born.

So we spent four days in the NICU working with lactation specialists and nurses trying to get her to eat and monitoring her waste. On Tuesday of that week, to our surprise, we came in the room to see her and found out that a nurse had given her a vitamin K shot without our consent. This proceeded to cause her bilirubin count to go up and she spent the next few days under a blue lamp or what they call a bili light to help rid her of the jaundice that she was now suffering with.

By Thursday night, she was eating and had gained a satisfactory amount of weight, so we were told that she would get to go home the next day. She came home on Friday afternoon and throughout the next few days at home she gained color and her expressive self returned. She got adjusted the very next day and has been receiving regular specific chiropractic care since. We have also chosen not to vaccinate her or give her any other shots besides the one given without our consent at the hospital. Praise Jesus, she is now a perfectly healthily and resilient kid.

I took my newborn to the hospital for what should have been a fairly routine heart rate check in the ER, but later turned into a myriad of medicals mistakes which nearly cost us the life of our baby girl AvaKate. Our situation with AvaKate unfortunately isn't an isolated problem. Medical research showed that 77 percent of medication errors in emergency departments occurred during the prescribing and administering phases, which is what happened with AvaKate. The most frequent error in these situations is the improper dose or quantity given, which has a 24percent rate of occurrence!

7.
Green Your Baby

Everything seems to be going green. From hybrid cars to hybrid fuels, detergent-free detergents, energy saving light bulbs, rechargeable batteries and on and on. I even get dirty glances at the grocery store if I don't bring my own bags. Everyone wants to be green about everything, except when it comes to food. Perhaps I'm exaggerating a little, but did you ever notice how people know more about where to recycle plastic and paper in their community than they do about the food and drugs they put into their baby's body? When was the last time most parents questioned what's in the milk or juice that their 6-month-old is guzzling, or the burger and fries their 20-month-old is chomping? If you're like me, those ingredients with "scientific" names in our baby's food just don't compute. It may seem like the "herd" is feeding it to their baby, so this food must be okay. This mentality is rampant amongst our families, schools and churches where our babies sometimes eat their snacks or meals. But I disagree. What exactly are all those extras that they put into the foods our babies eat? Have you looked at the ingredients list of those innocent little "Goldfish" crackers and read it? Do you realize what's in the bag or box your little one is drinking out of and how it has a shelf life of several years? Let's tackle some of the most common culprits in our baby's foods and expose the ugly truth.

The Bad and the Ugly

I could fill a book on the subject of chemicals present in the foods we feed our babies. The first culprit, high fructose corn syrup or HFCS, isn't really much different than plain old sugar, according to the most recent research. The reason that HFCS is used plentifully in hundreds of products you could buy at the grocery store is because it's much cheaper for companies to produce and use in their products than real sugar, which is made from sugar cane or sugar beets. High fructose corn syrup is an industrial food product that requires an enzyme process to bond fructose molecules to cornstarch, which basically means it's made in a lab and produced in a factory—totally man-made. HFCS is in many products we give to our babies, like breakfast cereals, mayonnaise, pancake syrups, jelly, ice cream and popsicles, crackers, yogurt, soda, breads, hamburger buns, juice drinks, snack foods, sodas and many more. Some researchers have questions about how our bodies process HFCS internally and make claims that long-term use could cause ill health effects. We think, let's just remove it from our baby's food supply and we won't have to find out about those possible long-term effects. But HFCS is tough to get out of our foods because it's in so many products. A good rule of thumb is that if the product is processed, chances are that it has HFCS in it. The only saving grace is that some stores like Whole

Foods, their affiliates, or some natural health food stores have corporate policies to either sell no products with High Fructose Corn Syrup, or to carry certain product lines with no HFCS in them. Buying any food that is designed by God for our babies, versus made by man, is the key to avoiding HFCS or any other artificial chemical. No one knows the long-term effects these chemicals have on our bodies and no research has been done on how they interact with babies that are breastfeeding or in early stages of development. When out of the ordinary diseases show up, the "experts" typically point to genetics in an effort to rationalize these diseases with unknown causes.

When at the supermarket, we attempt to abide by the adage of "shop the walls and not the aisles." In typical grocery stores, the outer walls of the store contain fruits, vegetables, poultry, nuts, meats, dairy, seafood and items that are more likely to be naturally fresh and very minimally processed. On the contrary foods in the center of the store, or the aisles, are the more processed foods in bags or boxes—the items with a longer shelf life. One more side note about sugar, for baby and the whole family, is that recent research from UCLA shows that depriving cancer cells of glucose (sugar) activates a metabolic and signaling amplification loop that leads to cancer cell death[1]. Cancer actually feeds on sugar, so we need to limit sugar intake, specifically the sugars found in processed foods. Too often, these sugars are also found in baby food or snack foods that most parents are feeding to their babies and children.

The second culprit is MSG, or monosodium glutamate. MSG is a man made ingredient used to alter our taste of

---

[1] http://newsroom.ucla.edu/portal/ucla/researchers-discover-that-glucose-235478.aspx

many processed foods and to trick our brains into thinking it tastes good. MSG is also found in hundreds of products at the grocery store, but many times it is a hidden ingredient because companies give it a different name in order to mislead us. These many different names include, but are not limited to: autolyzed plant protein, calcium caseinate, glutamate, maltodextrin, monopotassium glutamate, sodium caseinate, soy protein concentrate, textured protein, yeast food, and yeast extract, just to name a few. The list of possible names is enormous and the only way to avoid MSG is to avoid all processed foods, or to buy processed foods at a grocery retailer who will not sell MSG-containing foods in their store. High fructose corn syrup manufacturers wanted to follow the lead of MSG and be allowed to change its name to "corn sugar" to keep it as a hidden ingredient, so that the public wouldn't recognize it in their food. For now, this hasn't occurred. Because of the public outcry about the proposed change, the FDA would not approve "name changing" of HFCS. The research goes both ways on MSG, with some saying it's perfectly fine in certain amounts and other research stating that it is linked to a myriad of symptoms, many neurological in nature[2].

The third culprit is Aspartame. This chemical could and should be classified as enemy number one. Aspartame is a low calorie, artificial sweetener made from two amino acids, phenylalanine and aspartic acid. It is 220 times sweeter than sugar. You probably know its brand names, such as NutraSweet and Equal. Aspartame complaints account for approximately 70 percent of all complaints to the FDA![3]. It's in over 9,000

[2] http://rense.com/general52/msg.htm
[3] http://rense.com/general50/KILLER.HTM

products, including diet sodas, pudding, juices, children's vitamins, gelatins and on and on. Chewing gum is one I've noticed as of lately. Try to go to the grocery store or the convenience store and buy some gum without phenylalanine or aspartame. Good luck! Almost every gum you'll find has some form of artificial sweetener in it, specifically aspartame or it's derivatives.

Aspartame has been linked to serious disorders, such as behavioral problems (hyperactivity, aggression, learning disorders, poor learning ability and ADD) and a lifetime of endocrine problems such as menstrual difficulties, infertility and premature puberty. In clinical studies, it also complicates and worsens certain medical conditions like lupus, multiple sclerosis, Parkinson's, diabetes, retinopathies, allergies and mental disorders, etc. It has been shown to cause mental retardation, birth defects and many types of cancers, seizures, brain tumors and death. It's so toxic that a single ounce can kill or blind an adult.[4,5] It's safe to say that in our household, we agree to stay far away from aspartame, as we consider it to be the most deadly substance in foods. The majority of low fat or non fat food products contain these artificial sweeteners, as the FDA requires that all products put on the label if it has aspartame, Nutrasweet, Equal, or an artificial sweetener in it.

Nowadays, many people we come into contact with know the dangers of aspartame, but then they suggest Splenda as a good alternative to aspartame. This may be why Splenda has now replaced aspartame as the number one artificial sweetener

---

[4] http://www.laleva.org/eng/2006/09/aspartame_causes_birth_defects_and_mental_retardation.html
[5] http://articles.mercola.com/sites/articles/archive/2011/11/06/aspartame-most-dangerous-sub-stance-added-to-food.aspx

in foods and beverages. Dr. James Bowen, a researcher and biochemist, reports, "Splenda, or sucralose, is simply chlorinated sugar, a chlorocarbon. These chlorocarbons attack the nervous system and can cause cancer, birth defects and immune system dysfunction." The truth is that any sweetener that is artificially made, meaning man-made, will have side effects because of the way it's processed by the body. Splenda, otherwise known as sucralose, is added to many products, including many so called "health" or "natural" products. In fact, just the other day, a well-meaning and unaware practice member in our chiropractic office gave us a sample energy powder to add to our water. Unfortunately, we had to inform this individual that this "energy powder" contained the harmful ingredient sucralose and thanks but no thanks.[6] Due to the huge marketing effort by McNeil Nutritionals, Splenda has out sold all the other artificial sweeteners and become the number one artificial sweetener people choose.

Most of us would choose an artificial sweetener only because we believe it would help us cut calories and lose weight. We've been duped again. New research proves that people who drink diet soda actually gain weight. Researchers from the University of Texas Health Science Center (UTHSC) at San Antonio gathered ten years' worth of data on 474 participants from a larger, ongoing study called the San Antonio Longitudinal Study of Aging. Among these participants, those that consumed two or more diet sodas a day experienced waist size increases that were a shocking six times greater than those who did not drink diet soda[7]. Even further research shows that as-

---

[6] http://articles.mercola.com/sites/articles/archive/2000/12/03/sucralose-dangers.aspx
[7] http://www.naturalnews.com/033110_diet_soda_weight_gain.html

partame can cause infertility and all types of pregnancy issues. Dr. James Bowen says, "At every point in the fertility process, aspartame…. ruins female sexual response and induces male sexual dysfunction. Beyond this, aspartame disrupts fetal development by aborting it or inducing defects. And if a live child is born, aspartame may have damaged the DNA of the baby, cursing future generations." [8]

So, now you may be starting to think, Dr. Hess are you telling me to go live in the woods in a teepee and hunt and grow my own food, because that's the only way to avoid all this stuff? On the other hand, some people are prone to give up and think, I'll eat what I want and trust God with the rest. Neither of these extremes are a good idea. What we recommend is to become as educated as possible and make as many changes as you feasibly can while not crashing your budget. There will have to be some sacrifices to see changes, though. For example, if you're drinking diet soda or putting Equal in your coffee, you'll have to shift toward water instead of diet soda and buy stevia (a natural sugar) or other natural sweeteners instead of Equal, Splenda, or Sweet N' Low for your coffee. Living naturally and from the inside out for you and your baby is the right thing to do, but no one ever said the right thing to do was easy. Health from the inside out is a long-term approach. It takes time and repetition, preparation, some sacrifice and even sometimes refusal to follow the "herd," but it pays huge health dividends that you and your family deserve and that we believe God desires for us.

Pregnant or soon-to-be pregnant moms routinely ask us about what they should be eating while they are expecting.

---

[8] http://www.laleva.org/eng/2006/09/aspartame_causes_birth_defects_and_mental_retardation.html

With all the myths surrounding pregnancy, it can get confusing. Simply and honestly, we all should be eating the healthiest diet as possible at all times, regardless of whether we are pregnant or not, but we do understand what most are asking. Most people that ask us about our diet are eating the standard American diet of some healthy foods plus processed foods and fast foods, which have little to no nutritional value. Never a week goes by in our office that someone doesn't stop us mid-conversation to ask, "Drs. Hess, I just want to know. Are you vegetarians?" We find this question humorous because many in our culture seem to think that you have to be a vegetarian to look athletic or thin and be healthy. And no, we are not vegetarians. We simply try to eat as healthily as possible.

So, Drs. Hess, how should I change to make sure that my baby and I get all the nutrition we need? Like most people, our personal diet depends on our schedule, so with us and our schedule at the chiropractic office, we prepare and make all of our own food five days a week. On the weekends, if we eat out, it will be at the most nutritious and healthiest restaurants possible. In our case, living in Atlanta, there are more and more restaurants that offer many organic and natural food options and those are the types of restaurants we frequent. Understand full well though, that even at the most natural and organic restaurants you have to be cautious about what you eat. Since we enjoy cooking and preparing meals at home, we would never settle for a "subpar" restaurant that would be by some considered a "nice night out," but really is a chain restaurant where much of the food is microwaved, overcooked and full of antibiotics, hormones and chemicals. Most will think we are extremists, but just the thought of eating at so many of these places makes the food we prepare at the house taste all the better. While pregnant and nursing, as with anytime, we believe people should take the extra time and investment to buy, prepare and ingest only the most nutritious, natural and organic foods possible. Every situation is different; however, we can all make better choices and move in the direction of "eating to live."

Another challenge for women during pregnancy is the thought of gaining so much weight. In my case, I gained 42 pounds with Alyssa and 37 pounds with Gabriel. Everyone is created differently, just like a snowflake or a thumbprint, we all have our own development and pregnancy comes in all shapes and sizes, just the way God intended. How much weight should one gain is not a good question. You may ask, "If my weight is not within the parameters of what the "medical community" considers normal regarding weight gain, does that mean I am an unhealthy person or that I am not being a good mother to my unborn baby?" Every woman is uniquely created by God and every pregnancy is a different experience. As long as you are eating healthy, nutritious foods, your body knows what to do. It has that innate, internal intelligence that God gave each one of us. Being pregnant, however, does not give you the excuse to suddenly gorge yourself due to "around the clock cravings." In our opinion, "I just had to have a double cheeseburger with extra sauce, a large order of French fries and a milkshake," or a whole pint of ice cream is just a poor choice, not only for yourself, but also for your baby.

If you are having these cravings, then you need to analyze yourself and figure out what your body really needs. When I was pregnant with Alyssa, I craved citrus and lots of it. I ate oranges everyday and sometimes several times per day. Maybe I had a vitamin C deficiency. I don't know for sure because I didn't have any testing done to confirm this hypothesis—however, once she was born, I didn't want another orange for a long time. Everyone's pregnancy is different, but proper food and nutrition is a choice and it is your responsibility to make the right choices for your baby.

Our daughter Alyssa is six years old now and the foundation that we have set forth for her in her early years has paid off. If she is unsure if a food or beverage is healthy or organic, she asks us first if it is okay to eat or drink it. If there is a party at her school, we do our best to accommodate and provide alternative healthy snacks for her. She knows that eating and making healthy food choices is a priority for our family and that mainstream food is full of toxic chemicals and preservatives that will eventually be detrimental to one's health. Just the other day, she came home from summer camp to inform us that she told her best friend that drinking soda was not good for her. In my curiosity, I asked, "Alyssa, what did your friend say when you told her that?" Alyssa responded, "She told me that she would talk to her parents about this." That was a proud Mommy moment for me. I gave her a high-five and told her how proud I was of the good example she was setting for her friend.

With Gabriel and Alyssa, as they began eating solid foods at 6 months of age, we would go to Whole Foods market or our local natural foods co-op store and buy certain kinds of organic fruits and vegetables. We would prepare a significant amount of food for Alyssa or Gabriel all at one time for the next week. So for example, if it was avocado, bananas and butternut squash we were going to make for the week, we would bake the squash, put it into a small blender and blend until it was smooth in texture, then scoop it out and put some into small glass jars to put in the refrigerator, or into ice cube-type containers to freeze for use in the near future. Avocado and banana would be the same process (without baking them, of course) and the same goes for all types of fruits or vegetables we made.

As the kids have gotten older, we realize now that what we thought was a lot of work with making their baby food for the week from scratch was actually an easy task compared to the battle ahead of us with daycare, nursery and pre-K. In these programs, we have found that the administrators and teachers are all very well-meaning when it comes to being nutritious in their approach. The problem arises when these same people think that a morning snack should consist of Little Debbie snack cakes and a glass of whole milk, which contains growth hormones and antibiotics, or that it's okay to let the toddlers have cheap, chemically-laden ice cream every Friday from the ice cream truck.

Now, if you're in the fortunate situation where your toddlers stay home with you, then you can prepare the freshest and purest food for your little ones. If your kids are like ours where they spend Monday through Friday at a pre-k or elementary school, then you must learn the institution's policies on food and adhere to it, while still making sure your kids don't get caught up eating junk food all the time. We teach our kids to say no to anything the school might serve and we tell the school about our healthy food choices. We then explain to them

143

why we prepare and plan ahead. For example, the teacher will tell us a day or two in advance about a birthday party that is planned in the classroom, so then we send in something like gluten free, all-natural cookies for our kids to eat instead of party cake and ice cream. On ice cream truck day, we send an organic popsicle with our children to avoid the commercially made ice cream tainted with "chemicals" from the nice man in the truck. That way our children don't feel left out, but they also are not sacrificing their health.

It can seem like a battle when dealing with these issues and the truth is that at times it has been for our family too. But we live by the long-term approach, knowing and following the universal law of cause and effect. The types of foods and toxins or chemicals we put into our bodies and our babies' and toddlers' bodies will determine sooner or later the health outcomes that they have. Sometimes the effects might not be seen for months or even years, but there will be consequences for ignoring this universal law. In our society of fast pace and quick fix, the average person doesn't think twice about these kinds of things. They don't wonder, "Will my daughter start her menstrual cycle at eight or nine years old because of all the hormones she has been ingesting over her life?" or, "Do the constant antibiotics my children get in their food supply affect their immune system resistance?"

We didn't write this book for the average thinker and if you're reading this book right now, that means you're not average. You're above average in your desire to live your and your child's life as closely as possible to the way God intended. That's our "why" in writing this book, so that others could know there is a better way—a way that was designed by God.

Sean's Birth Story
By Naomi Rice

When my husband Jody and I first found out that we were pregnant with our first child, we were (of course) excited and overjoyed and I knew that I wanted to have a natural birth with as little intervention as possible. We attended an extensive 3 month childbirth class on the Bradley method for natural birth. During my pregnancy, I was blessed to find Doctors Jeremy and Amanda Hess. Not only did they help me have the best pregnancy, but they also provided a wealth of information and resources regarding information on such things as the truth about vaccinations, why babies should be checked and adjusted after birth and how chiropractic care can help pregnancy and labor. By the time I reached the end of my pregnancy, my husband and I felt fully prepared and ready to give birth naturally to a healthy baby.

We had arranged to give birth at the local hospital, but with a group of midwives who were completely on board with our birth plan. The hospital was not so prepared for us, though. My labor began at 41 weeks and we drove to the hospital when my contractions were five minutes apart. I was only 3 centimeters dilated, so we checked out of the hospital (which is not the typical procedure) and I continued my labor at my godparents' house. By the time my water broke, the contractions were still five minutes apart but much stronger and I had to completely relax during them. We went back to the hospital at this time and continued with labor for the next eight hours, although the time seemed much quicker than that to me. Jody and I had prepared and practiced this so many times that we had no anxiety or fear. He was my coach and advocate. While Jody straightened out paperwork issues, I talked with the nurses, who were very sweet. Whenever a contraction came, I politely said, "Hold on just a moment," closed my eyes and relaxed. Once the contraction was over, we continued our conversation. Jody passed out our birth plan to everyone who walked in the room so that everyone knew exactly what was going on, even if they were simply passing through. He also had to interact with the administrative staff because the paperwork they expected us to sign contradicted what was previously agreed to on our birth plan, so they had to compose new forms that were not contradictory. I'm so thankful that my husband took care of all that while I concentrated on laboring. Had he not been prepared for these obstacles, he might have signed and consented to the standard hospital protocols, which were in disagreement with our birth plan.

Throughout my laboring, news spread on the maternity floor that I was having a natural birth, so other nurses and staff randomly came into my room to pop their heads in to see what this was all about. One nurse told me, "Most of us have never seen a natural birth before!" I was shocked to hear this. Jody learned that at least 75 percent of the staff had never seen a natural birth; this explained why everyone wanted to stop by and witness it for themselves. I didn't mind, though. Prior to reaching the transition stage of labor, I enjoyed chatting with nurses and friends. As I bounced on a yoga ball, one nurse told me, "If you didn't have that machine to monitor your contractions, I wouldn't think you were in labor. You are much too calm and happy!"

When I reached transition, Jody read the signs and knew that we would be meeting our baby boy soon, so he encouraged me on through the toughest stage. Pushing the baby out was the easiest part. My body worked with the contractions (I was so thankful that I wasn't numb or drugged so that everything could work the way it was meant to) and I pushed through the pain, squatting on the table in the hospital room where we had dimmed the lights. Jody's excitement about seeing our son's head was a great motivation for the last two pushes and then our baby came right out, the pain was all over and I was holding our precious baby boy in my arms. It was the most wonderful feeling on earth! I immediately forgot about the pain that I had experienced and fell in love with this wet, wiggling little soul. He suckled my breast instinctively and we bonded for about an hour before I let the nurse clean him up, weigh him and hand him back to me. I was exhausted, as if I just completed a marathon (which I had, in a large sense), but I felt so content.

The birth of our son Sean, 8 pounds 5 ounces, was the most amazing, wonderful experience. After experiencing a natural birth, I cannot fathom ever even considering pain medication for this exhilarating experience. Sean was three days old when Dr. Hess came to our house after work to assess him for subluxations (bones out of alignment, a result of the birth process). Since his birth was so smooth and uncomplicated, he didn't need an adjustment, but as he grew, he regularly visited his chiropractor. Thanks to such excellent chiropractic care and a healthy lifestyle, he has never suffered from any ear infections, colic, major illnesses and has never been subjected to vaccinations.

8.
Correcting the Cause

It was a Monday afternoon at the practice, when we got a call from the nursery that Alyssa was running a temperature of 100.5 and needed to be picked up as soon as possible. With our busy schedule of serving hundreds of practice members per day at our office, these types of calls can be quite burdensome on us, but we knew what our daughter needed and it wasn't any fever-reducing aspirin or over-the-counter medication. Amanda went to go pick her up and Alyssa seemed somewhat okay, as many toddlers do with a low-grade fever—a little sluggish, but still acting normal in most capacities. Amanda brought her to the office and the first thing we did was to check her spine for vertebral subluxation, which is when one of the spinal bones misalign and cause nerve interference, resulting in dysfunction and/or dis-ease of the body. We wanted to make sure her spine was in proper alignment so that her nervous system could function at its best and her little body was at its optimum to fight whatever kind of virus or bacteria that it had encountered.

Before we continue Alyssa's story, let us explain further that if you've parented any children, you know that these situations can happen quite frequently. On a daily basis we see babies and children in the office that are brought in by their parents with a fever, whether it is a 100.5 or a 103.5 and the parents have learned that a specific chiropractic adjustment will help optimize the immune system response of the child and naturally assist in lowering the fever. Many parents view fever with fear and anxiety due to the implications of possible febrile seizures and brain damage if the child gets too hot; however, God created fever as the body's natural sign that it is fighting an infection.

In toddlers a fever is a very common response to the teething process or their body having an episode with a virus or bacteria. Whatever the fever is from, after we perform a gentle specific adjustment, usually in the upper neck area at the atlas vertebra (the first vertebral bone of the neck), we always tell the parent to check the child's temperature within two to three hours. Typically, one of two things happens. Either the fever spikes momentarily and then reduces as the body's natural response takes over, or the fever reduces within that time frame. Parents will come in on the next appointment for the child and say, "Just like you said Dr. Hess, the fever was virtually gone in two hours."

Now on this occasion with Alyssa, the fever was not gone in two to three hours, actually she felt hotter than she did before. We say felt because we've never used a thermometer, simply because we believe the body's innate intelligence will never harm itself, but will always protect itself and do everything possible to keep the system functioning normally. This is not to say you shouldn't have a thermometer—you should do whatever your comfort level is, but don't over react with "thermometer syndrome".

Afternoon led into evening and then bedtime and Alyssa was still with fever. She seemed to sleep fairly well, though she woke up a few times and we kept her hydrated with water. The next morning, she was burning up. We had quite a week. We look back now and see how God was testing our faith in many things, one of them being the principle of inside-out healing. Did God really give our little girl an innate intelligence that had everything she needed to fight this fever or was it going to be necessary to use pharmaceuticals or other medical treatments? Everyone has to face their fears and that week we faced ours. Alyssa didn't eat anything that next morning or even that next day. She went four days without eating anything except liquids and ran a fever for five days with one night where she was up all night. During that night we were hydrating, checking her spine and certainly praying over her. We were on the brink of giving in. We would look at each other, Amanda in tears and say, "This principle of healing and chiropractic from the inside-out works for every other child God—why not ours?"

That week we learned the true meaning of the phrase "Feed your faith and starve your doubts." We didn't give in like everybody else we know and give her fever-reducing medication or run to the pediatrician. We stood our ground together and stayed faithful and we were victorious in our battle. It also helped that both of us were on the same page regarding our daughter's health. So many times we hear from friends and practice members that one of the parents, or better yet, a grandparent pressured the child's parent to take the child to the pediatrician or urgent care. With our family, Amanda and I are congruent, so there was never an argument about Alyssa's situation and what we should or should not have done. Looking back now, we are thankful for those five days. They further strengthened our belief system and Alyssa's immune system will forever be stronger because of them.

What's your reality? Is your baby or toddler consuming antibiotics at an ever-increasing rate? Does your little one seem to "catch" the bug, cough or cold that comes along through daycare or the nursery? We care for many babies and toddlers that come to see us with all types of ailments, including ear infections, asthma, colic, constipation, immune disorders and other "all to common" infant conditions. Many of these conditions will amazingly resolve themselves without any intervention and gentle specific chiropractic adjustments assist in the healing process naturally.

Ear infections, which are the number one reason parents take their toddler to the pediatrician, are a perfect example of a common infant problem that needs little or no medical intervention. The AAP (American Academy of Pediatrics) says that most of these infections are just middle ear fluid and it recommends a "watch and wait" approach and no treatment. Of the small percentage that actually are a classic ear infection, or "acute otitis media," the AAP says that 80 percent of these cases will get better without antibiotic treatment. Numerous medical journals since the mid 1990s have all pointed to the ineffectiveness of amoxicillin and other antibiotics for ear, sinus and respiratory infections, even to point out that in almost all cases the antibiotic prolongs the infection and can set the stage for reoccurrence. Yet while pediatricians see millions of toddlers every year, they continually prescribe them antibiotics like amoxicillin, even though their own medical research says not to do so.

Maybe your toddler just seems to be symptomatic all too frequently and you are taking him to the pediatrician's office every few days or weeks getting rounds of antibiotics and shots or being frequently poked and prodded. The good news is that for these babies and toddlers, there is a better way! Research shows that routine specific and scientific chiropractic adjustments boost the immune system and allow an infant's body to function the way God intended, healing naturally from the inside out, without drug intervention.

Our society is plagued with ideas, concepts and beliefs that slant toward a quick fix or a cover up of the symptom instead of getting to the root cause of problems. It is widespread in people's relationship issues and in their emotional, mental and physical problems. Even on a spiritual level, many times we're guilty of seeking God only in a crisis, as if to ask God to cover us when there is a storm or "crisis" in our lives. Divorce rates are 50 percent or more, mental health issues are escalating and physical stress has hit all time highs.

When it comes to physical health, we would like to enlighten you on the most magnificent, amazing and powerful healing potential of all time. It has the ability to heal all your diseases, whether physical, mental, emotional, or chemical. It can ward off cancer, mend broken bones, conquer asthma and allergies, clear up your chronic sinus problem, break the cycle of infertility and so much more. How much does it cost? Where do you find it? Why has no one ever told you about it?

The great news is that it's free! You received it as a gift and God gave it to you when you were conceived in your mother's womb. It's called the innate intelligence of your body.

Innate means that it was inborn, planted by God inside your very being to regulate, coordinate and direct all your bodily functions. The innate intelligence didn't need to be told how to develop your heart and start it beating, or to know that you needed ten fingers and ten toes. This inborn intelligence created the millions of filaments in your eyes and miles and miles of blood vessels that travel the course of your body. It makes your body shiver when you get cold and sweat when you get hot. It produces a fever if you're fighting an infection, or diarrhea if you ingested something toxic. This inborn wisdom was with you in your mother's womb and is still with you today, performing millions of internal mechanisms every second without ever having to think about it.

Now, unbeknownst to us, the educated world that we live in starts to tell us over time that our babies' bodies, their innate intelligence, is inferior, that it needs help from an external source to regulate and direct the body's functions. It says that your baby needs an aspirin to fight the fever or a flu shot to help ward off the flu, as if God didn't give your baby everything it needed when it was born. Some of these ideas that our babies are lacking comes from the medical paradigm and Big Pharma also drives some of them into our minds. Either way, these belief systems lead to intervention after intervention and only lead to further long-term damage of our babies' health.

Either way these belief systems lead to intervention after intervention and only lead to further damaging our babies' health in the long term. The core essence of our mission is to teach people a process of striving to live their lives from the inside out. It's the way we live and have programmed ourselves to think, to look at our habits and the actions of ourselves and our children. We evaluate things not from a worldly perspective, one that has a "herd" mentality, but a vantage point that God gave us everything we need and it's on the inside of us. We are created in His image, made complete and whole in Him.

We both grew up in good homes that emphasized having a good work ethic, doing what is right and respecting our parents, other authorities and God. Both of our parents are still married after 40 years and they gave us and taught us everything we needed to have a good life. As we look back now, regarding health, both of our childhoods involved very little medications and doctor's visits. It may have been our parents, who were cautious of too many drugs and medical intervention, or the culture of the mid 70s and early 80s, when the use of drugs was much more focused on "street drugs" and the "Just Say No" campaign." We did, however, both get all our vaccines per the schedule at the time and our parents followed the routine medical protocol regarding checkups. Thankfully during our childhood, the number of vaccines given was less than a third of the vaccines currently recommended and the toxicity in foods, water and air was minimal 35+ years ago when compared to the levels exposed to this generation. This generation of children is being attacked from so many different directions and their health and longevity are taking a big hit! We believe there is a better way and making sense of these complicated health situations is our top priority.

Noah's Story:
A baby's painful tears
becomes a family health testimony

By Mindy Silva

My husband and I had never been to a chiropractor before and we never really even gave it much thought. Noah was our third child and at six months old, he started having ear infections. For six weeks, he had a double ear infection. During the next eight weeks, our pediatrician put Noah on seven different prescriptions. The problem, however, was that the pharmaceuticals made him even more sick, stripped his immune system and never even cleared up his ear infections. With the ear infections still occurring, the doctor told us the final option and necessary intervention would be ear tube surgery. Like many other parents, we trusted Noah's pediatrician that he was giving the best advice based on his knowledge and if the tubes were going to fix everything, then we were all for them. So, we got tubes in his ears. We were shocked when just two weeks later after the surgery, he had another ear infection! Once this happened, Noah's pediatrician referred us out to many other doctors for his ears. After all the antibiotics and surgery, we still had no solution and we were spending a lot of money on pharmaceuticals and doctor's visits, not to mention a lot of painful crying for Noah and mommy. This went on for six additional months with more medications and many sleepless nights for Noah and mommy.

On Noah's one-year-old birthday, which should have been a joyous day for him and our family, he took a turn for the worse. He became severely sick with a double ear infection and a very high fever of 104 degrees. The doctor sent us to the hospital for him to have blood work done and receive more shots. In fact, he had a total of four shots, one shot daily for four days. That night my husband and I broke down and fell to our knees praying over Noah for God to help us. The next morning, my mother called and told us she found Discover Chiropractic and Drs. Hess. I was unsure of chiropractic and had no clue that chiropractors could even help a one-year-old, but I said as long as they did not poke needles at Noah or give us more meds, I was ready to try anything. My husband and I had never been to a chiropractor before and just went based on my mother's advice and really as a last resort. My mother kept encouraging me, so I scheduled the appointment. When we arrived after a 45-minute drive, Drs. Hess' assistants immediately made me feel welcome and encouraged. They took the time to explain how chiropractic could help Noah, as well as help the entire family. I left that appointment feeling encouraged, uplifted and hopeful. When we returned to Drs. Hess' office for our second visit, we sat in a new patient class, where they explained how God designed the body, health and healing the natural and chiropractic way and health and healing the allopathic or medicated way. The presentation left me in tears as they were explaining the natural versus medicated road of health. Flashbacks of everything about my Noah was going through my head from the past year.

We started going three times a week for three weeks, which was quite the commitment considering how far away we lived. But it was so worth it. During that first month, Noah was sleeping better and suffered no ear infection. After four months going twice a week, still no ear infections. After a year, NO ear infections! Noah is two-and-a-half years old now and still healthy.

Now our whole family is under specific chiropractic care and we thank God every day for healing Noah and giving Drs. Jeremy and Amanda Hess a gift of helping people.

Our health is forever changed! Thank you!!

Rhyder's Birth Story
by Robyn Sabo

For as long as I can remember, I always knew I would have my babies at home. I am not sure where this desire came from but it was always within me, God-given I suppose. I never welcomed the thought or idea of being interfered with during labor, although I had no idea what labor and birthing would be like, as I had never attended a birth.

Prior to having children, I was in excellent physical shape. I had been a gymnast as a child and teenager and was very strong compared to others. My core especially was always very strong. I was fit. I thought I was healthy; I ate well, studied nutrition and took relatively good care of myself.

However, prior to getting pregnant, I had been on birth control for over five years. I had begun to find myself very emotionally unstable and through trial and error of eliminating different foods and stressors from my life, I came to recognize (with the help of my husband) that I was experiencing side effects from my birth control. I was emotionally a wreck, depressed and unpredictable in how I coped with life.

We decided it was in my and our marriage's best interest to discontinue the birth control. After stopping the birth control, which I now realize caused artificial hormone changes within, I suffered severe acne all over my face for the next year and a half. It was like my body was reacting to no longer tricking it with hormones and beginning to heal itself by releasing all the birth control toxins through my skin. It was a tough year and a half looking at myself in the mirror, but time and the body's innate healing took care of it. I look back now and am thankful that it only took a year and a half to purge from my system, since I had ingested over five years' worth of birth control.

A year and a half later, I was pregnant for the first time. My first pregnancy seemed typical. The only part that bothered me constantly was that as the baby developed, I was extremely sore all the time and often felt quite uncomfortable. I bled often throughout the pregnancy, which caused a constant fear of miscarriage. I went from exercising five to seven times per week to nothing, for fear I would bleed more or worse, lose the baby. I had major yeast infections during this pregnancy, which was strange because I had never had one before being pregnant. The worst part, however, were that my feet were literally covered in warts from the bottom of my toes to the middle of my foot. The entire ball of my foot had hundreds of warts. I didn't try to overanalyze the situation; I just chalked it up to being pregnant! My midwife concluded that the physical discomforts I suffered had to do with me being a former gymnast with extremely tight ligaments and muscles. The rest of my immune system issues, however, couldn't be explained, aside from hormone changes.

After 13 hours of intense, constant and very difficult labor, my daughter was born naturally at home with no epidural or pain medications. It was not what I had anticipated and dreamed of, but my midwife's words stuck with me. She had always said throughout my pregnancy that "we sometimes don't get the delivery we want, but we always get the delivery we need." I didn't quite understand that, but I knew it was significant. I was thrilled to have a homebirth because I knew that in a hospital setting, due to the length of time of my progression and labor, I would have been just another woman under Pitocin at the hospital's mercy, artificially monitored and told when to push, resulting in fetal distress, with my daughter being forcefully pulled out with assistance, like forceps or vacuum. My midwife said that in a hospital, they may not have allowed me to push for as long as I did and that a Cesarean may have been the outcome. It always saddens my heart for all the women who never get to experience natural childbirth, but have the false misconception that the doctor saved them and their baby when the reality is that one intervention only leads to the next intervention.

My daughter was nearly nine pounds and my recovery afterwards was long. I recall beginning an exercise program four months later and nearly falling over from discomfort after doing a squat. My hips felt terrible and my entire bottom felt like it was tearing apart.

I now realize that each person is an individual and each person heals differently. It took a long time—what seems now like forever—but eventually my body healed and I returned to my pre-pregnancy activities. I also relied on chiropractic more than ever before to assist my skeletal structure and help my immune system rebound. I always remember the chiropractic statement that "proper structure equals proper function." I was able to return to my pre-pregnancy fitness level by the end of my first year post-partum. My warts went away within a month of giving birth and I no longer suffered from yeast infections.

Two years after having my first child, I felt normal again, but not perfect yet.

During that time, I learned more about chiropractic than I had ever known before. I got checked and adjusted regularly instead of when I felt I needed to. I came to understand that my nervous system was interfered with and needed to have that interference removed so that I could function at a higher level of health.

I then got pregnant with my son and carried him completely differently than my daughter. I carried him straight forward, like a torpedo! I also had him at home. My hope was that I would be able to say my labor and delivery was amazing; it was easy and it was everything I had dreamed it would be. I was told by so many people that it would be better because it was my second one. My midwife reminded me, "You will get the birth you need and I can't tell you it will be what you expect."

My labor and delivery was two hours shorter than my daughter's; however, it was perhaps more difficult than the first go around. My son was born face up and the delivery was tiring and hard. I had a healthy, smaller baby at just seven pounds, which most people would think would be much easier, but the opposite was true. My midwife reassured me that my body was made for birth and that I had to trust that nature knows best. My husband assured me that the inborn intelligence that God had put in me knew what needed to be done in order for my son to be born. It was no mistake that I had a big first baby and a small second one. My daughter paved the way for my son to enter this world naturally without any interventions. I hear of so many women who are induced because they are seemingly carrying a "big baby" and God must have made a mistake because their pelvis is too small to birth their baby. I feel women are falsely made to believe that their bodies aren't perfectly made for birth and they are feared into induction and intervention.

After birthing our son, I continued on my chiropractic health journey over the next two years. I was even more consistent with care. My chiropractic adjustments were done specifically and scientifically to correct the interference in my body. Although the delivery was difficult with my second, my recovery time was incredible. I did not experience the hip and pelvic pain like I did with my daughter's recovery. Instead, I felt like I was ready for baby number three right away! My husband thought I was nuts, but that was how much better my body was functioning. Two and a half years later, I found myself pregnant again with my third baby. I also carried this child straight forward, but this baby felt heavy. I gained the same amount of weight as with my son; however, my belly felt full. I was big! I was so big that I got a lot of attention from friends, family and strangers all the time. It was unbelievable.

My midwife kept reassuring me that everything was okay. With all the attention, this couldn't be normal. Was this baby huge? What exactly was going on? I would constantly ask her. Later on, after my delivery, she shared with me that she was concerned I was going to have difficulty delivering this baby because it measured big. So, just in case, she brought two additional midwives along just in case there were complications. I am so glad that she didn't share her concerns with me prior to the delivery. Her positivity and extra cautionary measures kept me at peace so that I never doubted my body's ability to birth.

The delivery was nothing short of ironic—I had my primary midwife and two additional midwives for this delivery, but this time, I got the birth of my dreams. It was four hours in length from start to finish. My water broke and I went into labor within the hour. The labor continually progressed as I paced the hallway at home and I labored and delivered in the pool. No birth is easy, but this time it was manageable. It was consistent and continued to progress. I did not struggle or become weary or fatigued. My son, Rhyder, was born without any complications. The extra midwives had nothing to do. In fact, they went home before I even understood why they were there. My primary midwife continued to monitor me and when the time came to weigh Rhyder, we all stood there in amazement as the scale bounced well beyond nine pounds and he weighed in at 10 pounds, 5 ounces.

Rhyder's birth was by far the best, easiest and most empowering birth ever. My body was ready; it was properly aligned and prepared through regular chiropractic care and this time, nerve interference was no longer an issue. My pregnancy was amazing. Despite the size of my belly, I was able to run well into my eighth month of pregnancy. I did not have the discomfort or stretching pains and I did not experience hip and pelvic discomfort at all. I never experienced any infections or complications with my nervous system like I did during my first pregnancy.

When people tell me that their doctor told them they are too small to have babies, I disagree. I know that birth is not always easy. It is definitely not enjoyable, but it is possible! I do believe that some women are so structurally interfered with that delivery becomes impossible under standard expectations. I also know that the body is capable, if it is given the right time and has had the interference removed. I have had three children: a big baby, a fairly average sized baby and a huge baby! The biggest one was the easiest pregnancy and delivery. Size has no influence. It's the level of interference in your body that makes the difference.

By the time I had my third child, I had been under regular chiropractic care for over six years. I had to work through a lot of interference and stress to get to the point where birth could be uncomplicated. Everything works together and there is a reason for everything. I now know that with time and repetition, my body healed and my small frame was able to deliver a large baby with no difficulty at all. Specific, scientific chiropractic care made all the difference.

9.
Our Stories

Jeremy's Story

It was an amazingly sunny day in Topsail Beach, North Carolina and I was 13 years old and determined to be a better boogie boarder than my two older brothers. As the day progressed, the flips and crashes got more and more dramatic and by days end I was my own self-proclaimed expert. Unfortunately, I had to pay the price of showing up my brothers, so the next day I woke up and could hardly move my neck. As the day progressed I started feeling strange sensations with shooting pain down my right arm. By that evening my mother had me off to a local medical office to get evaluated and I was quickly given muscle relaxers and sent home.

Over the next 24 hours the pain in my arm started becoming more frequent and with every painful grimace on my face my mother grew more concerned. To my mother's surprise, my dad mentioned that they should take me to a chiropractor, so off we went and I got my first ever chiropractic adjustment. Unfortunately, I never had a follow-up appointment with this chiropractor and since I was out of pain, my parents saw no need in taking me to a chiropractor back home in Westchester, Pennsylvania. It wasn't until 4 years later when I was travelling once again that I received my next chiropractic adjustment.

I was 17 years old and while fishing in Alaska, my buddy and I decided to sleep in a pick-up truck. I awoke to horrendous pain. I would later learn the technical term for this condition: torticollis, an abnormal, asymmetrical head or neck position. Basically, my neck was twisted and I couldn't move it myself back into a normal position. This time around, however, I knew exactly what to do. Unfortunately, I was in the middle of nowhere in Alaska. I told my buddy, Jeremiah, that we had to find the nearest chiropractor. He thought I was crazy, but he complied.

After one chiropractic adjustment, I felt much better and ended that trip with that chiropractor taking us fishing on his personal boat! I returned home once again without seeking a follow up with a local chiropractor, because I was still living in the medical model: "If there's no pain or symptoms, then everything is fine and that means I'm healthy." Or in other words, "if it ain't broke, then there's nothing to fix." A year went by and while playing collegiate soccer, I injured my hip during a game and was sent by the team's coach to the medical doctor to receive muscle relaxers. As God would have it, one of the players on the team had close family connections with a local chiropractor.

As I hobbled into his office I noticed something different compared to the previous chiropractors I had encountered. There seemed to be a different feeling about the place. There were lots of people coming and going and not just people in pain. Most looked like families with children who obviously were not hobbling around like I was. After I was evaluated and X-rays were taken of my spine, the chiropractor came in to greet me. He analyzed my diagnostics and I returned for my much needed chiropractic adjustment. After four visits to this chiropractor, all was well and I was back playing again which was vitally important since I was on a partial college soccer scholarship.

About two weeks after meeting this chiropractor, he offered to take me to lunch where he explained to me the healing principles of chiropractic and how the body was made to heal and function from the inside-out. It all made sense to me now. I even began to put other puzzle pieces together, too. While under the care of this very proficient chiropractor, not only did my hip improve, but I also recognized that I hadn't had to use my asthma inhaler anymore. I was also able to throw away eye drops I had been taking for over two years due to a chronic eye infection that inexplicably never had cleared up—until now. This one lunch was definitely a God moment for me, as I decided shortly after that lunch to visit Life University, school of chiropractic. Within six months, I was moving to Atlanta, Georgia, to attend chiropractic school.

Jeremy Hess, DC

Amanda's Story

On a warm autumn afternoon in Columbia, South Carolina, I lost my balance and fell from the top of the cheerleading pyramid. This fall ended with Heidi's knee in my back as she caught me. The pain was immediate, so I left practice and went home. By the time my mother came home from work, the inflammatory process had taken over and I was crawling on my hands and knees. My mother helped me to the car and we drove to urgent care. I remember receiving a shot in my back and I was given pain pills, muscle relaxers and anti-inflammatories and told, "everything will be okay."

I've talked to so many people over the years in this same situation. My problem was that "everything was NOT okay!!!" I was in severe pain, couldn't get comfortable sitting and I was not cheering or attending my dance classes. As a sophomore in high school, this was unacceptable. At that time of my life, dancing was my passion. I was dancing at least five days per week and competing in various state and national competitions throughout the year.

The pain made me desperate. I would do anything to get out of the pain so I could return to dancing as soon as possible. It just so happened that my ballet instructor at the time was married to the local chiropractor. My father was positive about seeing the chiropractor. As an avid golfer and a winner of both the State Amateur and Senior Amateur golf tournaments in South Carolina, he frequented his chiropractor when in pain or in need of a tune up with his golf game. I remember entering Dr. Frost's office, getting some spinal X-rays and lying down on the table, thinking that whatever he was going to do—whatever this so-called chiropractic adjustment was—it couldn't possibly make my situation any worse. As he was making my spinal adjustments, I was surprised at how the bones moved, the noises they made and then finally thrilled to get off the table feeling pain relief for the first time since my initial injury. Dr. Frost gave me follow-up appointment recommendations beginning with appointments three times per week and it gradually lessened over the course of time. Unfortunately, I never truly understood the importance of continued chiropractic care even when out of pain. Being the teenager I was at the time, I got busy with school and extra-curricular activities. Since I was free of pain and dancing again I stopped going to see him.

I graduated high school as salutatorian of my class and pursued my Bachelor of Science degree in biology at the University of South Carolina (go Gamecocks!). During my collegiate years, I was a research assistant at the local hospital in the molecular genetics department for bone marrow transplantation. My father and everyone I knew expected me to attend medical school, become the next great medical doctor and bring honor and prestige to the family. One afternoon at the hospital changed my life. I was exiting the elevator like I had done hundreds of times before, but this time was different. As I was walking through the lobby, there was a family huddled together, weeping and sobbing. It was very clear they had just lost a loved one to cancer. I left work that day with tears in my eyes thinking…

- Is what I am doing really making a difference?
- Are we really ever going to find a "cure" for cancer?
- Do I want to work in a hospital for the rest of my life?
- Do I want to be the person to tell a family that their loved one is not going to live?

Over the next few months, I halfheartedly completed my biology degree. I finished college confused, acknowledging that I didn't want to be a part of the medical community for the rest of my life, but not really knowing what I should do. I informed my father that I wasn't going to apply to medical school, which was a major letdown for him. I decided to move to Atlanta, Georgia, where I was alone and jobless. I spent the following year working as a server at various restaurants and meeting a lot of great new people. Many of them attended Life University, a college of chiropractic.

One of my co-workers was in her clinical experience of chiropractic school and asked me if I wanted to become one of her patients. The cost was rather inexpensive and since my prior chiropractic experience was great, I thought, why not? So, I began to receive regular chiropractic care again. During the course of my care, I realized that chiropractic was my answer. I could still help people with their health, but in a very different way, a way that would give life. Chiropractic was (and still is) the answer to restore health to someone's life. I applied to Life University and the rest is history.

Jeremy and I met in chiropractic school, fell in love and decided to make this our life mission... well, not quite! To the surprise of everyone, however, our romance did not start in chiropractic school, but in a parking lot in Buckhead, a well-known area of Atlanta. I was a restaurant server at a popular fine dining restaurant to pay my bills and Jeremy was parking cars to pay his bills. We said a few words to each other here and there, but never had much time for conversation, as we were both on the job. One cold rainy night, however, Jeremy ran across the parking lot to ask me for my phone number. I gave it to him and then in disgust watched him write it down on one of the $20 bills he had earned that night. He said he would be calling me and I just walked away thinking, "Does he think I am that much of an idiot? He just wrote my number down on a $20 bill!" Needless to say, he called, our relationship developed and we were married on a beautiful spring day in April 2002.

Words cannot express how much Jeremy has influenced my life on a personal, spiritual and chiropractic level. As someone who first went to the chiropractor for pain (as most typically do), I thought that was all there was to it. Since Jeremy was graduating with his Doctorate of Chiropractic degree at the same time I was entering the program, he had already learned the true magnitude of a healthy functioning nervous system and had witnessed amazing healings through chiropractic. Every chiropractor has a moment, one specific chiropractic adjustment that changes their life forever. For me, I was fortunate that my moment occurred early on in school.

One summer evening, this older couple that Jeremy had been taking care of for a number of months had extra tickets to a local concert and invited us along. Before the concert we met them for dinner at a local steak and seafood restaurant. Jeremy ordered the seared tuna and I ordered the salmon; dinner went well and then we went to the concert. By the end of the concert, Jeremy began to complain that he was hot (I thought nothing of it—Georgia is hot in July, so just get over it!). We left the venue and headed home, but Jeremy kept saying how he didn't feel well. He asked for me to pull into the office parking lot, as it was on our way home and he proceeded to run inside to the bathroom.

As I followed him and stood outside the bathroom I proceeded to listen to him have diarrhea like I had never heard in my life—it sounded like the faucet on the sink had been turned on. As he was attempting to compose himself, I felt his forehead. It was burning hot. Then he said he felt itchy. His arms had red dots all over them. Then we unbuttoned his shirt and his chest was covered with them as well. I didn't know what was happening. Was he dying? Did I need to call the ambulance? This was definitely a medical emergency.

Jeremy, however, had a clear enough mental capacity with all this going on to say, "Amanda, calm down. My innate intelligence is getting rid of whatever is affecting me—that darn tuna fish. I think though I am out of alignment and I need you to adjust me." I said, "Jeremy, I am only in the beginning of school. I have only taken a couple of classes. I don't know what I am doing." Then he quickly told me what to do, gave me a couple practice runs and said, "You can do this," and laid down on the table. I placed my hands on his neck, adjusted him and stepped back in silence. Jeremy just laid there and said nothing. Time seemed to stand still in that very moment. He then sat up and said he was feeling a little better but wanted to lie down a bit longer. After that one adjustment, his diarrhea ceased and within 15 minutes his skin rash had almost completely resolved. That evening was when I truly realized what one simple yet specific chiropractic adjustment could do for someone's health.

Amanda Hess, DC

10.
A Different Lens

It all seems so normal now for us to view life, health, disease and the body through the lens of a natural inside-out chiropractic perspective. We know it's a very different lens and viewpoint than most people living in the Western world, but we believe it's a much more accurate, scientific and godly perspective.

Chiropractic works with the innate intelligence of the body, that inborn wisdom that God gave each one of us when we were conceived. We believe that God does not create junk, but created us in His perfect image and thus the body has everything it needs and doesn't require interference. Instead of looking at the body and studying everything that's wrong with you—all your diseases, symptoms and health problems, we prefer to focus on what's right with your body by evaluating and applying the principles of health, life and longevity to have your body express its full God-given potential.

Our job is not to treat or suppress your symptomatology—on the contrary our goal (and the goal of specific chiropractic) is to correct the underlying cause of the problem and to restore life to your body, allowing your body's innate intelligence to fully express itself and your body to function normally. Chiropractic does this by working closely with your nervous system, which is the master control system of your body.

Your nervous system, which is comprised of your brain, spinal cord and millions of nerves in your body, allows for proper communication from your brain to all parts of your body. A chiropractor's main focus is to locate, find and correct any spinal nerve interference between your brain and your body, as this spinal nerve interference can disrupt the body's normal function and cause damage, dysfunction and ultimately disease if left uncorrected. Spinal nerve interference is more technically known as vertebral subluxation complex, which simply means you have a spinal misalignment or vertebra (spinal bone) out of proper position causing nerve interference.

Chang Ha Suh, PhD, a spinal biomechanics expert at the University of Colorado, found through extensive research about the spine, vertebral subluxations and nerve interference, "Subluxation is very real. We have documented it to the extent that no one can dispute its existence. Vertebral subluxations change the entire health of the body by causing structural dysfunction of the spine and nerve interference. The weight of a quarter on a spinal nerve will reduce nerve transmission by as much as 50 percent."[1] This reduction in nerve function is what we aim to correct with the hundreds of practice members we encounter everyday in our practice. We care for all types of people with all types of problems ranging from babies that are just a day or two old to someone that may be well into their nineties. Chiropractic restores proper nerve function through

[1] http://sitochiropractic.com/nrp.html

specific chiropractic adjustments, all the while utilizing a scientific approach with space-certified technology that measures nerve interference to accurately pin-point and obtain an exact assessment of any problem areas a person may have, regardless of their condition of disease—or even if the person has no disease or problem and appears to be heathy.

German medical research performed in the 1980s examined a random group of 1,250 babies five days post-partum (after birth) and showed that 95 percent of these babies were found to have abnormal stress or strain in their neck region with 211 of them suffering from vomiting, hyperactivity and sleeplessness. Gentle chiropractic adjustments of this group frequently resulted in immediate quieting, cessation of crying, muscular relaxation and better sleep.[2]

Another German medical researcher found 80 percent of all children are not in structural balance and that many have subluxation and nerve interference in the upper neck and atlas region at the base of the skull. The research summarized that even with the lightest adjustment with the index finger, the clinical picture normalizes, sometimes gradually, but often immediately. This research found that common complaints such as tonsillitis, conjunctivitis, frequent colds, ear infections, sleeping issues and intestinal problems all were resolved through gentle specific chiropractic adjustments.[3]

You may be thinking, "Why has no one ever told me this before?", or "I wish I would have known this when I was raising my children and they were sick all the time." That's what we

---

[2] http://mychiro4kids.com/ciropractic-for-kids--why.html

[3] http://icpa4kids.org/Wellness-Articles/your-inner-wisdom-trusting-the-process-for-natural-birthing/Page-2.html   http://wwwchiropractic4al.com/reports/kidschiropractic.htm

hear far too often on a daily basis in our practice when we educate our practice members on the wonders of chiropractic and how the body can function best when the nervous system is free of interference. It's exactly why our children, Alyssa and Gabriel have been cared for with specific chiropractic care since they were in Amanda's womb and due to chiropractic, lifestyle habits and the grace of God neither of them have ever taken any pharmaceuticals, whether over-the-counter or prescribed. The good news is that your babies and toddlers can be just as healthy as ours and grow up as drug free children, just like Alyssa and Gabriel. Remember, God gave us everything we need; we just need to utilize the knowledge, take action and have faith that there is a better way.

Fevers, headaches, stomachaches, strep throat, ear aches, coughs, colds, sneezes, asthma and allergies are just a short list of the things that can affect your bundle of joy. There have been times when Alyssa or Gabriel have been "sick" and "symptomatic" with fever, coughs and sneezes, or they have gotten the "cold" that's going around. All of our little ones will suffer with some of these ailments and even the ones with the best immune systems become victims at times.

The question becomes not whether they will get symptomatic, but what will your reaction and thought process be when they do? The first thing to understand is that the majority of symptoms in infanthood are normal reactions of the body fighting infection or warding off some type of toxin. Secondly and the most important point, our body is always striving for homeostasis, or balance. Your baby wasn't designed to be sick, but actually designed to be balanced, whole and healthy.

Asthma

160% Increase in Children Under the Age of 5 Since 1980

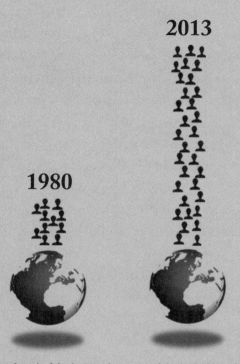

2013

1980

According to data from the federal agency that compared the 1997-1998 and 2007-2008 time periods:

- Average annual percentage of American children treated for asthma increased from 4.7 percent to 6.1 percent.

- Average annual prescription drug expenses for a child with asthma more than doubled, from $349 to $838.

- Children ages 5 to 11 years were more likely to be treated for asthma than children ages 12 to 17.

- Overall average annual health care expenses per child with asthma increased 37 percent, from $1,827 to $2,503.

The data in this AHRQ News and Numbers summary are taken from the Medical Expenditure Panel Survey (MEPS), a detailed source of information on the health services used by Americans, the frequency with which they are used, the cost of those services, and how they are paid. For more information, go to Statistical Brief 332: Health Expenditures among Children with Reported Treatment for Asthma, United States, 1997-1998 and 2007-2008.

The symptoms that your baby or toddler express are really its attempt at regeneration and healing. A book that we give to all our practice members who are expecting a baby and a must read for any parent with children is, *How to Raise a Heatlhy Child in Spite of Your Doctor*, by Robert S. Mendelsohn, M.D. It's a fantastic book on all types of childhood ailments, how to determine if and when your child needs to see a pediatrician and a common sense medical approach to keeping your child healthy, drug-free and out of the doctor's office.

We've both been receiving regular specific chiropractic care for over 20 years. Trauma is one of the main ways that any of us can become subluxated or go out of spinal alignment and cause the process of nerve interference that deteriorates our health and well being. Amanda has had her fair share of bad car accidents living in Atlanta, numbering five total with most causing her severe neck pain and headaches, not to mention the countless years of repetitive trauma caused by dancing and cheerleading. Jeremy has two older brothers to blame for many of his head and neck injuries, which are evident in a history of multiple stitches in the front and back of his head , on top of years of battling it out on the soccer field playing defense. Our son, Gabriel, is a classic example of "all-boy behavior" jumping off stairs, doing flips on the couch, sliding down slides backwards, or worse yet, sliding head-first instead of feet-first. Just the other week, he crashed his bike with bruises and scrapes on his hands and knees.

Doing things repetitively is another prime example of how subluxation or nerve interference of the spine can occur. When Alyssa was three years old, she started picking up our cell phone, watching and playing all sorts of kids' games. Think about our toddlers and their propensity towards electronics and computers and the repetitive stress it can cause at such a young age on the neck and upper back structure and muscle tone. For hours each day, our babies are also in car seats or in a seated position, which is not a normal posture or skeletal position. All of these daily traumatic events and repetitive activities lead to interference within our nervous system.

In the early stages of these interferences of our spine, many times there are no symptoms, but when left uncorrected over time, symptoms and degenerative changes will ultimately occur. It is always the same response when we ask parents if they take their children to the dentist. They always say, "Yes, of course we take our kids to the dentist." The next question we ask is, "Why do you take your kids to the dentist? Is it because their teeth hurt or are in pain?" Then the parent responds, "No, their teeth don't hurt. We want to make sure everything is okay and that we prevent them from having any cavities." Our response is, "Well, then why wouldn't you take your children to see a chiropractor to make sure everything is in proper alignment and prevent any type of neurological or structural damage to the spine?" It is unfortunate that most parents never have the opportunity to be educated on the importance of regular chiropractic check-ups for their children. One thing we always remind each other and our practice members is that we are changing the world one spine at a time. That's our mission—to help families be healthy and understand the necessity of a properly functioning nervous system.

Pregnancy can also be very trying on a mother's spine, with the typical busyness of today's society keeping her working and playing right up to the birthing process. With all of a pregnant woman's demands, there is a tremendous amount of lifting, bending, pulling and twisting. Research shows that when a pregnant mother receives regular chiropractic care throughout her pregnancy, she experiences 84 percent less pain throughout the pregnancy, her labor time during birth decreases by 24 percent and in cases of women who have had multiple births, their labor time is reduced by 39 percent.[4] Chiropractic adjustments help realign the pelvis, allowing for less pain and complications during the birth process.

During the birthing process, most mothers get into a situation where they are in a compromised position, lying on their back in a hospital bed and unable to move. Remember, the baby should be descending out of the birth canal, where a mother would be delivering in a squatted position or a kneeling position, which is normal.

The traditional hospital birth requires the mother to go against gravity, due to lying on her back and the baby ascending out of the birth canal. This type of birthing actually dates back to the seventeenth century and King Louis XIV. The king wanted to view his maidservants give birth, so he would have his maidservants be placed on their back and give birth, while he would hide behind a curtain where he couldn't be seen. The rest is history, as birthing has kept that ritual to this day. The laboring mother lying on her back is a great position for the doctor or nurses, because they don't have to get on their hands and knees or in awkward positions as the baby crowns and is delivered.

[4] http://www.planetc1.com/chiropractic-articles/pregnancy-chiropractic.html

Unfortunately for the laboring woman, this has caused a great degree of problems and need for intervention in birthing. While the mother is lying on her back, the weight of her own body and the baby causes excessive pressure on major blood and nerve centers, such as the abdominal aorta and lumbar spinal plexus. This disadvantageous birthing position, potentially stressful medical environment and invasive drugs can all lead to a "traumatic birth." A traumatic birth is caused by any excessive force used to deliver the baby out of the mother's womb. Manually pulling the baby out with obstetrical forceps, vacuum extraction, or C-section delivery all cause extremely abnormal force on a newborn's head and neck. This pulling, twisting and rotating can cause the baby's first vertebral subluxation and spinal nerve interference in the upper neck, which is exactly why every newborn needs to get checked and evaluated by a chiropractor to see if there is any nerve interference present.

Getting your newborn checked within the first week of life and having the chiropractor gently and specifically remove any nerve interference allows the baby's body to be healthy and function normally. We have been checking and adjusting our two children since they were both just a few hours old and they both get weekly chiropractic checkups to maintain their health and vitality. Everyday, we are so grateful for the knowledge of chiropractic and the wisdom of allowing the body to heal from the inside out and that our children and the thousands of children we have taken care of over the years are living proof that God truly gave us everything we need, Now you and your baby can achieve the health that you've always wanted and been praying for, because there is a better way!

Kirk's Birth Story
By Theresa Stover

My first birth was a wonderful experience. I had no epidural or medications with the birth of my daughter, Becky and I was expecting to do the same with my second child.

With the second birth, we planned a birthing room so that our five year-old daughter, Becky, could be part of the experience. I went into labor naturally and all was going as expected. When contractions would come we would breathe through them and Becky would feel the tightness of my belly. She and my sister-in-law sat on the couch reading little golden books and drawing pictures for the new baby.

Things were going just fine until I got to the point where I wanted to begin pushing. Now this is where I should have gone with my God given natural instincts and not the "wisdom" of the medical experts! I asked the nurse to get the doctor so that she could check me. At that present moment the doctor was sleeping, so the nurse proceeded to tell me that she herself had just checked me 10 minutes prior and I was only at 6 centimeters and only 70percent effaced and there was no way that my body was ready to start pushing. She refused to get the doctor and did not examine me, but she did proceed to tell my husband that if I "couldn't handle the contractions at 6 centimeters there was NO WAY that I could handle them at 10." Then she began FEAR statements like: "SHE needs to rethink not having the epidural because her daughter is in the room and if she doesn't get it now then she'll have to do this without anything and the baby may go into distress", etc. etc.

Well, you could imagine the emotions and fear, the concern and fear, the anguish and fear and did I mention the FEAR!!! At this point my husband and I talked and decided that yes, we should do the epidural. Remember during this whole time I kept feeling like I needed to push, but the nurse kept telling me not to push.

So they called in the anesthesiologist who administered the epidural without anyone checking me for dilation or effacement. The epidural then kicked in and that is when my troubles began. As it turned out, my son WAS in the birth canal and I **should** have been pushing. Well, because of the epidural, my contractions stopped. The doctors and staff got very frantic and inserted forceps to pull him out. One nurse was above me pushing on my belly as the doctor was pulling. They succeeded in pulling him out, but I didn't have my next contractions to expel the placenta. The placenta tore and I lost 4.8 pints of blood. First, they packed me with packing gauze to try to stop the bleeding. They tried this 3 times with no success. They also tried manual manipulations of my uterus and abdominal muscles. This was extremely painful and caused bruising that took several weeks to go away.

At this point the doctor turned pale and expressed to us the dangers if I didn't stop bleeding. She called in a surgical team to take me in for an emergency hysterectomy. I just laid there crying, confused and scared. We asked the doctor what else could be done. All she said was, "Get everyone you know to pray." They removed the packing, put me at the end of the bed with my legs up in stirrups, placed a 25 gallon bucket on the floor under me to catch the blood and the surgical team stayed lined up at the wall watching over me, ready to pounce!

The sound of each drop of blood hitting the bucket was the scariest sound my husband and I have ever heard. We felt so hopeless. We laid there holding hands, praying and crying. Then God answered our prayers. In exactly 29 minutes the bleeding stopped and, I never had the hysterectomy, but I also couldn't have any more children because ¾ of my uterus was scarred from that event.

Twenty years later, Becky still remembers bits and pieces of that day. Some people say that history repeats itself, however, to avoid another natural birth gone wrong, Becky chose to have both of her children at home and the most rewarding part of these birthing victories is that I was there supporting her.

Kylie's and John Mark's Birth Story
by Becky Harrison

Even before my husband, Mark and I were "man and wife", we talked about our family, the one we hoped to have one day. We asked questions like how many children do we want, do we want boys, girls and how long do we want to wait to start a family once we get married. But most importantly to me, we asked how and where we planned to birth our babies. I had grown up with a fear of hospitals because of my mother's incident and I knew there had to be an alternative. My husband was equally leery of hospitals after another nurse's error almost caused his own grandfather to bleed to death internally.

Almost a full year before I got pregnant, I found a website about a midwifery service and the woman I knew I wanted as my coach. Along with choosing to have a home birth, Mark and I also chose not to have any of the typical medical procedures associated with pregnancy and birth, like routine ultrasounds and other tests.

My pregnancy was perfect. I followed my midwife's advice. I charted my eating habits to stay accountable. I exercised and did yoga at home. I walked a 15-minute mile 3 times a week. I took my prenatal vitamins. I obtained regular chiropractic care, which effectively eliminated the "usual" low back pain, headaches and morning sickness that most people associate with pregnancy. I was also able to do many things you wouldn't expect a pregnant woman to be able to do, like take karate and work right up until the day I went into labor!

At one of my many visits, my midwife gave me a worksheet and she asked that Mark and I use it to write out what we imagined as the perfect birth. Here is what we wrote: "I imagine my birth will be at dawn or dusk, when the lighting is naturally low, a peaceful—yet painful—time. We would like to have classical music or nature sounds playing softly, the lighting dim." We went on to list our preferences such as who in our family we'd like to have present at the birth, that Mark would like to catch the baby and cut the cord and how we'd like to spend the first moments after the baby was born.

After a day of sporadic contractions, Mark and I spent the evening at home watching a Star Wars marathon and eating Subway sandwiches. Around 9 pm, we called the family to let them know what was going on and told them we'd call again whenever we thought the baby was coming. Around 11:00 pm, the contractions were still about 15 minutes apart and lasting just 20-30 seconds. My midwife told us she could come to our house, but that if she came too soon, I might feel pressured to "do something" and my labor could stall out. I thought, "That sounds a lot like what happens to women when they first rush to the hospital thinking they're in labor only to then not have their labor progress by standard medical protocols.", So we decided to wait and call again when I felt ready for her to come to our house.

At 4:46 am, Mark called our midwife because I could no longer talk through my contractions. She asked to speak to me. I was barely able to utter a "hello?" and she said "I'm on my way!"

Mark called the family and told them all to "come NOW!". At 5:15 am my water broke.

When Joy, our midwife, arrived, she told Mark to go ahead and start filling the pool for the waterbirth. He told her he didn't think there was time. She then did her initial exam checking my blood pressure, my heart rate and baby's heart rate.

At about 5:50 am, I said, "Oh, it hurts!" That's actually the first moment I had an almost—but not quite—unbearable pain. Joy said, "I see the top of the head, that's why it hurts so bad. Your baby is almost here!" Mark made his way from my side, where he had faithfully stayed and held my hand as each contraction got harder, to the end of the bed just as yet another contraction hit. I clenched my jaw to hold back the pain and my mom rubbed my face and said "don't clench your jaw, baby". As she rubbed my face, I consciously made the effort to unclench my jaw as the next contraction hit at 6:00 am, this time bringing the entire baby with it! Joy wrote in her notes "4 contractions from first glimpse of baby's head to birth!"

Because the baby came so quickly in so few contractions and it was born holding its fist to its face, I did have a pretty major perineal tear that required stitches. The suturing was actually the most intense pain of the entire process because while your body creates hormones to help you cope with the pain of delivery, there are no hormones created while getting stitches!

The placenta was delivered and we waited until the cord stopped pulsating before Mark cut the cord, in order to allow all that blood left in the placenta to transfer into the body of our newborn baby. Then, we spent 15 minutes, just the 3 of us, as everyone had quietly left the room to give us some privacy.

Then Mark and I looked down under the towels, then back at each other and grinned as we announced, "It's a GIRL!"

Once we announced the gender, my baby girl and I went for our celebration bath where a warm bath was drawn, special healing herbs were added to the water along with the tops of a bouquet of flowers that my younger brother had brought to us. It served a few purposes: it allowed for a very gentle cleansing of the newborn baby, the herbs used would help speed the healing process of my tears and the pictures we were able to capture during the bath are priceless to us.

Kylie Nicole Harrison was born at home at 6:00 am without any medical interventions whatsoever. My total labor from the beginning of Stage 1 (when my contractions became consistent) lasted just 7 hours and 46 minutes. I had no monitors, no medicine for the pain and I would do it again in an instant.

After the "perfect" birth of our daughter, my husband, Mark and I agreed we would definitely go with a homebirth again. So, when I had another positive pregnancy test a couple months after Kylie's second birthday, we called our midwife to schedule prenatal appointments.

As with Kylie, I again had a great pregnancy. Everything went smoothly until I was 34 weeks pregnant. I was driving to my chiropractor with Kylie one Saturday morning for our regular check up when I was in an extremely bad car accident. I was hit in the rear driver's side and it spun my car around; then I was hit again in the front driver's side which spun the car around again. The impacts caused all the side and driver's airbags to deploy, the driver's airbag hitting me right in the chest. I immediately started having contractions that were just 5 minutes apart and I called 911.

The ambulance arrived and I was thoroughly examined. Thankfully my contractions stopped after about 40 minutes. The EMT's asked if I would like to be taken to the hospital and I declined. See, in my state, as in many others, homebirths are frowned upon by the "medical community". I was honestly afraid that the medical personnel at the hospital might treat me badly because I hadn't done all those tests that they think are so important and they would want to subject me and my unborn child to a slew of what I feel are unnecessary procedures. Now, you may be reading this and you may think, "Surely doctors or nurses would NEVER treat a patient poorly for refusing a test, right?" So why then did I feel this way? Well… my own OB/GYN refused to see me during this pregnancy because I had planned a home birth!

After refusing treatment at the hospital, I called my midwife and my chiropractors, Drs. Hess, to let them know I was in an accident. Dr. Jeremy said he would come back to the office that evening even though they were supposed to be closed so Kylie and I could be checked and adjusted. Then after much advice, I agreed to have one ultrasound done to make sure the placenta was still intact and fully attached to the uterine wall. It turned out that everything was fine. Due to the fact that this was considered a "high risk" situation, getting the ultrasound made sense.

Just 10 days before my due date I started having those "different" contractions I had experienced with Kylie. I called my midwife just to inform her and we agreed it was early labor. By 2:00 pm that next afternoon they were about 10 minutes apart, but they still weren't very strong so I called with just an update. By 7:00 pm they were seven to eight minutes apart, though they were still not very intense. Knowing how quickly labor progressed with Kylie, Mark and I agreed we should go ahead and call Beth, Rachel and our families to have them come on to the house. Beth arrived at 9:05 pm. She checked my blood pressure, my heart rate and baby's heart rate and everything looked great.

Unfortunately due to all the excitement, my labor stalled out and I went from having contractions every seven to eight minutes to about one per hour by 11:00 pm, so Beth sent almost everyone home. Mark woke up at 5:00 am on Thursday and asked if I thought he should stay home or go to work. I told him to go on because I hadn't really had any contractions. He went to work and I went back to sleep.

Not even two hours passed and I woke to an intense contraction. I didn't think much of it until I had another contraction just six minutes later. At 7:00 am I called Mark to come back home and I called Beth to come back to my house.

By 10:00 am, everyone had arrived and I was sitting in bed, able to talk, laugh and play with my daughter until a contraction came and Kylie would breathe deeply along with me and rub her little hands on my belly while she talked to the baby.

At 12:30 pm my water broke. I got into a semi-sit position on my bed as that was what felt most comfortable to me. Mark helped prop me up with pillows and Beth coached me through several pain-coping techniques. During this part of my labor as the pain from the contractions and from the baby being in the birth canal got intense, Beth suggested that I reach down to feel my baby. I could just feel the top of its head and I remember telling Mark to feel the baby with me. I remember talking to the baby saying things like "We're a team", "We're working together little one". Mark even said, "Come on little one! Mommy and Daddy can't wait to meet you!". I kept my hand on my baby and visualized it coming through the birth canal. With the next few contractions I could feel more of its head, then its head and shoulders and at 1:06 pm I actually "caught" my baby myself and pulled it up to my chest! I saw immediately as I was pulling the squalling baby to my chest and announced, "Oh, you're a BOY!"

Thanks to Beth's recommendations for preparing myself and my scar tissue from the tears I received during the delivery of Kylie, I did not tear very badly at all with my son. The placenta was delivered effortlessly just minutes after my son and his cord stopped pulsating. Then Kylie put on her bathing suit and got into the tub with "her baby" and me for our celebration bath once again.

John Mark Harrison, III was born at home at 1:06 pm, with no medical interventions. My total labor lasted just six hours and 20 minutes. Again, as with Kylie, I had no monitors, no medicine for the pain and I would do it all over again.

11.

Premature Birth to an Early Grave

My people perish from a lack of knowledge.
Hosea 4:6 (KJV).

So many parents have a sheer lack of knowledge on many of these subjects we've talked about and shared. They are in the situation that they simply don't know that they don't know: "The doctor never told us that." This is why we are on a mission of reaching the world with the message of inside-out health and healing and conveying the message that our bodies were truly designed by God.

This is a message that there is another way.

But we live in a quick fix, hurry up and suppress the symptom society, which covers up the problem and puts a blanket over the fire.

Our society does this rather than looking to the cause of the symptoms, or understanding that the expression of symptoms may actually be a good thing and in many cases, those symptoms are a wake-up call to change lifestyle habits

In this day of information overload, how could anyone be short on knowledge, or be lacking the vital information to keep their baby completely healthy and to make the best choices for their little ones? The truth is that we are not short on information. Google and Bing are a click away; it's just the source of the information that is the problem. Most health-related information on TV or the web is coming from pharmaceutical drug company sources. Marketing pharmaceuticals at us and our children is what drug companies do best. We are so susceptible to bending an ear to hear about the latest drug that might solve our baby's current ailment or illness and we quickly look to the medicine cabinet or a doctor for advice on the next miracle drug or treatment.

For Dr. Stephen Borowitz, a professor of pediatric gastroenterology at the University of Virginia, the most frustrating office visits are with parents of kids suffering from stomach aches and infants prone to spitting up. Often, he says, the parents already know what they want—adult heartburn drugs, such as the "purple pill," Prilosec. "I tell them about nondrug tactics that often help the symptoms," says Borowitz, "But they want their kids to have the pills they've seen on TV."[1] This is a classic situation that happens thousands of times a day in pediatricians' offices all across America.

Most of us grew up this way, with a medicine cabinet in the bathroom and our parents giving us a drug when we had a headache or stomach ache, yet they taught us that "street" drugs were bad. Most of our parents were probably somewhat cautious of how many over-the-counter and prescription drugs

[1] http://www.motherjones.com/politics/2003/09/doping-kids

we took. As most of us can remember, drugs are what we took for what ailed us, while at the same time, Nancy Reagan was on TV touting how we needed a drug-free America. If you're about our age, which would be a kid born in the 70s, you remember the 1980s TV commercial where they would put an egg in a frying pan and narrate: "Here's your brain (the egg) and here's your brain on drugs (the fried egg in the frying pan)." The announcer would then ask, "Any questions?" This is how most of us remember our childhood years, full of news reports about street drugs and how harmful they were and the "scared straight" program, scaring kids away from taking street drugs.

In the 70s and 80s the general public consensus and mindset toward taking a pharmaceutical was, "I have symptoms and an illness, should I take a drug?" Since then, the general mindset has changed to, "I have symptoms and an illness and instead of "should I take a drug?", it is now "which drug should I take?"

In a matter of 20 years, big pharma has changed the public's mindset from thinking about taking a drug as a solution, to taking a drug being the only solution. It's a very profitable mindset shift for the pharmaceutical industry. "Something like a third of consumers who've seen a drug ad have talked to their doctor about it," says Julie Donohue, a professor of public health at the University of Pittsburgh, who is considered a leading expert on this subject. "About two-thirds of those have asked for a prescription. And the majority of people who ask for a prescription have that request honored."[2]

As Bill Maher says, "*Tell your doctor...*" *Tell your Doctor? Shouldn't your doctor tell you what drugs you need? If you tell your doctor, isn't he just a dealer at that point?*"

[2] http://www.npr.org/templates/story/story.php?storyId=113675737

Until recently our children were a vast untouched market for the pharmaceutical industry. The drug companies had captured the older population because senior citizens would do anything their doctor told them. Slowly, the pharmaceutical companies have taught the baby boomers to rely on medications as a first choice and they now have lured us to believe that even infants and children need a constant supply of medications and shots if they are to stay healthy and well.

Ann Smith, Medco public-relations director, notes that recently prescription spending for children rose faster than spending for any other group, including seniors and baby boomers.[3] We see it all the time in our chiropractic office as parents bring their babies and children in for a specific chiropractic adjustment. They start by telling us about how the doctor said that the child might have an ear infection, early onset of asthma or strep throat and all too quickly hands out antibiotics, steroids, or some type of prescription. The parents blame the doctor for always giving a drug and in some cases, the doctors point the finger at the parent for demanding the drug and, if they don't get it, threatening to go elsewhere. Either way, the children take the hit and their health suffers, their immune system gets suppressed and they eventually end up losing.

Just when we think that the tide is turning towards natural health methods and the public mindset is shifting towards health and healing God's way from the inside-out, some new drug hits the market and the pharmaceutical industry pushes harder in the other direction. Make no mistake about it; as more parents get informed, big pharma will push harder in their marketing

[3] http://www.dailypaul.com/270147/vaccinated-children-five-times-more-prone-to-disease-than-unvaccinated-children?page=1

efforts. In the Atlanta metro area, where our chiropractic office is located, there has been a huge push for increased awareness of vaccinating babies and children. Why is this so? Well, the CDC (Center for Disease Control) and vaccine manufacturers have seen that the unvaccinated rate in Georgia has been climbing as in many other states. The most absurd advertisement, found on many major roads in the Atlanta area, are billboards depicting an "oh-so-cute" baby with the line: "No shots!" …. "No kisses!"

Unfortunately, most parents are uninformed and will never be told about the research pointing to unvaccinated children being healthier. They actually will be scolded by their pediatricians or even, dismissed from the doctor's practice if they don't get their children vaccinated. The American Academy of Pediatrics is now teaching pediatricians to pediatricians to guilt and fear parents into vaccinating their children if a parent happens to question a "normal" vaccine schedule or, God forbid, considers not vaccinating their child.

In an excerpt from *Pathways* magazine, one article elaborates on this point:

> Part of the "promotion of the positive value of vaccines" include The American Academy of Pediatrics website materials instructing pediatricians on how to handle parents who refuse to follow the CDC vaccine schedule. Excerpts from a sample letter states: "By not vaccinating your child you are taking selfish advantage of thousands of others who do vaccinate their children, which decreases the likelihood that your child will contract one of

these diseases. We feel such an attitude to be self-centered and unacceptable... Furthermore, please realize that you will be required to sign a "Refusal to Vaccinate" acknowledgement in the event of lengthy delays.

Finally, if you should absolutely refuse to vaccinate your child despite all our efforts, we will ask you to find another health care provider who shares your views. We do not keep a list of such providers nor would we recommend any such physician."[4]

We hear from countless parents who may have questioned the safety of vaccines, or who marvel at the sheer number of vaccines given now, as compared to when they were kids. Despite this questioning, however, they are told that their children had to get the shots or else they wouldn't be allowed in school. In Georgia, though, there is an exemption—in fact, all states have either a medical, philosophical, or religious exemption. For more information on your particular state, just go to www.nvic.org.

The next comment by the parents is always, "Our pediatrician and/or the school nurse told us that it was required. In fact, we asked them. Are you telling us that they have lied to us?" We have to answer that while we wonder if the pediatrician or nurse knows the law (which they should). "Perhaps they are just not informed of what the law is. We're sure he or she wouldn't misinform these parents intentionally."

Even a little research on this subject and its potential merits (or lack thereof) is perplexing. While much of medical research done in the United States points to all the health benefits of vaccination, the majority of the research on vaccines outside the U.S. points to unvaccinated children being healthier. Look at these two examples, the first from a pediatrician's office official statement—which was reprinted in the American Academy of Pediatrics News:

We firmly believe in the safety of our vaccines. We firmly believe that all children and young adults should receive all of the recommended vaccines according to the schedule published by the Centers for Disease Control and the American Academy of Pediatrics. We firmly believe, based on all available literature, evidence and current studies, that vaccines do not cause autism or other developmental disabilities. We firmly believe that thimerosal, a preservative that has been in vaccines for decades and remains in some vaccines, does not cause autism or other developmental disabilities. We firmly believe that vaccinating children and young adults may be the single most important health-promoting intervention we perform as health care providers and that you can perform as parents/caregivers. The recommended vaccines and their schedule given are the results of years and years of scientific study and data gathering on millions of children by thousands of our brightest scientists and physicians.[5]

[5] http://aapnews.aappublications.org/content/29/5/26.2.extract

Are they serious? Do they really think that thimerosal (mercury, a heavy metal) in vaccines is not a problem? Do they really believe that vaccinating your child is the single, most important "health-promoting" intervention they do? It simply startles us that these so-called health experts aren't even aware of the research being done about vaccinated children versus unvaccinated children and the results of those studies.

Pull back the blinders and start doing a little research yourself. Our suggested reading in the back of the book will help you become more informed if you desire, but check out this recent research:

An ongoing study out of Germany comparing disease rates among vaccinated and unvaccinated children points to a clear disparity between the two groups as far as illness rates are concerned. As reported by the group Health Freedom Alliance, children who have been vaccinated according to official government schedules are up to five times more likely to contract a preventable disease than children who developed their own immune systems naturally without vaccines.

Released as its own preliminary study back in September 2011, the survey includes data on 8,000 unvaccinated children whose overall disease rates were compared to disease rates among the general population, the vast majority of which has been vaccinated. And in every single disease category, unvaccinated children fared far better than vaccinated children in terms of both disease prevalence and severity. In other words, the evidence suggests that vaccines are neither effective nor safe.[6]

[6] http://aapnews.aappublications.org/content/29/5/26.2.extract

We honestly believe that one of the goals of the pharmaceutical companies is to establish our children as life long customers. There is no profit for big pharma if our children are healthy and drug free. There also is no profit if our children are dead, but there are hundreds of billions of dollars to be made on our children if they can teach us that our children need drugs and need them for a lifetime. Look at the latest horrifying statistics: "These days, the medicine cabinet is truly a family affair. More than a quarter of U.S. kids and teens are taking a medication on a chronic basis, according to Medco Health Solutions Inc., the biggest U.S. pharmacy-benefit manager with around 65 million members. Nearly 7 percent are on two or more such drugs, based on the company's database figures for 2009.[7]

If that did not shock you, you need to re-read those last two sentences! 25 percent of our kids are taking pharmaceutical drugs on a chronic basis! Are we the only insane or abnormal parents who think this is not okay?

The increase in childhood disorders is also astronomical and alarming. Dr. Kenneth Bock, co-founder of the Rhinebeck Health Center, has stated that as of 2007, ADHD (Attention Deficit Hyperactivity Disorder) is up a whopping 400 percent over the last 25 years. Bi-polar disorder has had a 40-fold increase among children over the last decade. Since the 1980s, asthma is up 160 percent in children under the age of 5 and autism has also had dramatic gains, with an estimated one in 88 children in America today having an autism spectrum disorder. 40 percent of children now have allergies. 25 percent of children have sleep disorders, which is also a precursor linked to obesity, asthma and allergies.

---

[7] http://online.wsj.com/article/SB10001424052970203731004576046073896475588.html

ADHD
Attention Deficit Hyperactivity Disorder

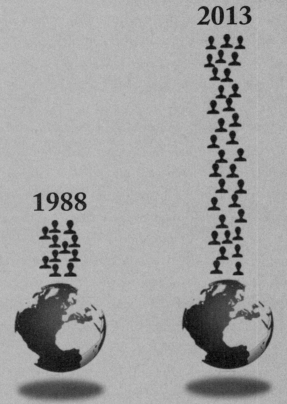

2013

1988

400% Increase Over the Last 25 Years

FDA records show that, between 1999 and 2003, 78 million prescriptions were written for ADHD drugs for children ranging in age from one to 18. A review of adverse events posted on the FDA website reveals that, between January 2000 and June 30, 2005, there were nearly 1,000 reports of psychosis or mania possibly linked to ADHD drugs, with psychosis characterized by the inability to distinguish real and imaginary events.

-Dr. Kenneth Bock

Co-founder of the Rhinebeck Health Center and author of (*Healing the New Childhood Epidemics: Autism, ADHD, Asthma, Allergies*) (Ballantine Books, 2007).

Moreover, researchers have found that every additional hour per night a third-grader spends sleeping reduces his or her chances of being obese in sixth grade by 40 percent. Nine hours and 45 minutes of sleep seemed to be the magic number of sleep hours for a third grader.[8] These figures are hard to believe, especially if your children are fairly healthy or don't take any prescriptions, but the fact is for every healthy child, there is another that is desperately sick and being treated medically from the outside-in.

If we as a culture continue the unnecessary medical treatments and drugs, bad nutritional habits and lack of proper life enhancing protocols—like specific scientific chiropractic care, providing proper organic whole foods and positive God-filled uplifting environments for our babies and children, then we can only expect these trends to continue and get worse.

As we sit idly by and do nothing, many of our babies and children continue to become a statistic, "With more children taking more adult drugs, often in combination, dangerous side effects are on the rise. Between 1997 and 2000, the FDA received more than 7,000 reports of adverse reactions to drugs in infants and children under the age of two, according to a University of Maryland study. Most of the reactions were serious enough to require hospitalization and 769 of the children died.[9]

When we were growing up, you didn't hear about peanut and milk allergies in every classroom, or kids having ADHD, asthma, learning delays, weird autoimmune disorders, childhood cancers and so on. This is quite the epidemic now. Some health professionals would say that our diagnostic abilities have just

[8] http://fixithealth.blogspot.com/2007/11/are-our-kids-sickest-generation.html
[9] http://www.motherjones.com/politics/2003/09/doping-kids

improved, but doesn't common sense tell everybody that these numbers aren't adding up? The amounts of sickness, disease and behavioral problems have skyrocketed and the numbers aren't getting better; they continue to rise. We say it is time to rise up and wise up to what is really happening to our precious children.

Why does it seem like the vicious cycle of symptom, drug, symptom, drug keeps happening to so many of our babies when we take them to the pediatrician? The big issue is how we view health and sickness. We have all been taught to believe health comes in a bottle and that any symptom that our baby or ourselves have is bad and needs to be suppressed immediately. So we do what our well-meaning parents taught us and what the pediatrician or nurse says and we continue patching up our baby's "sickness" or symptoms.

For example, when you give a baby with acid reflux a medication like Prilosec or Prevacid, essentially you're covering up or suppressing the symptom, which ultimately will cause other health issues for the baby. Think about it—what would you do if your car's oil light came on, meaning that your oil needed to be changed?

We're sure you would drop by an oil lube place and get it taken care of, because you know what could happen if you didn't. But just say you didn't have time or didn't feel like it and you ignored it, or better yet, you got a piece of duct tape and put it over the oil light so you wouldn't have to see the light anymore! What would happen! Your engine would soon start to smoke, then it would eventually seize up and stop working!

Thankfully you could always get a new engine, but what about your baby who you've given the acid reflux drug to? Isn't it like putting a piece of duct tape over the problem and ignoring the cause of the problem? "In a commentary published in *The Journal of Pediatrics*, Eric Hassell, MD, a pediatric gastroenterologist at Sutter Pacific Medical Foundation in San Francisco, warns that the use of acid-suppressing medications to babies under one year old has skyrocketed. One large study in the U.S. found a 16-fold increase in the number of prescriptions for a kid-friendly liquid form of acid-suppressing drugs between 1999 and 2004."[10]

This research article and others say that in most cases the problem will resolve itself over time and too many drugs are being given and often times because the parents demand it! With this infant health issue like so many others, dietary changes and specific chiropractic care along with time and natural remedies will correct the underlying cause of the problem and avoiding things such as vaccinations, pharmaceuticals and harsh chemicals found in foods is a must.

Unfortunately, pediatricians downplay the seriousness and potential danger of drug side effects; some medical personnel even outright dismiss them.

However, babies are much more likely than adults to react adversely to drugs. Some of the drugs you might think of as relatively safe, such as aspirin, over-the-counter cough and cold medicines and anti-nausea medications, are the biggest culprits. Even worse, many doctors get kickbacks and money from drug companies. Research shows that pharmaceutical salespeople can influence doctors on prescribing habits, with 8 out of 10

---

[10] http://www.webmd.com/parenting/baby/news/20111020/are-too-many-babies-getting-acid-reflux-drugs

doctors admitting to accepting free samples, gifts, or payments from drug companies. To see a list of doctors on a national database that lists doctors who are receiving drug kickbacks, go to: http://projects.propublica.org/docdollars. We must begin to realize that medical care and drugs are best used in emergency care situations. This is what they were originally designed for and emergency care only represents a small fraction of the overall health care industry.

Over the past six years with our son and daughter, we have had only one incidence of necessary medical intervention due to an emergency situation. Our daughter was playing and running along the concrete outside our office. She slipped on the air conditioning condensation on the ground and fractured her elbow. We proceeded to Children's Healthcare of Atlanta to X-ray and confirm the fracture. We then scheduled a follow-up visit with the orthopedist who casted her arm for the next six weeks.

A questionable part of this story occurred when the cast was taken off her arm. The doctor proceeded to examine the arm and elbow, check the range of motion and ask our daughter how it was feeling. Everything appeared okay, there was no swelling or discoloration, she moved her arm fine without any pain and she was happy to have the cast off, but he still recommended a follow up X-ray to make sure that it was healed.

When he said this, immediately, my maternal instincts said to me, "Amanda, is this totally necessary? She appears to be fine—this just doesn't feel right and I really don't want to radiate her if it is not necessary." So I looked right into his eyes and said to him, "Doctor—with all due respect I know that I am not a qualified orthopedist, but if this was your child, would you get the follow up X-ray? Everything appears to be fine. What do you think?" He responded, "Ma'am, if this were my child, I probably would not get the follow up X-ray...But that is the protocol for everybody."

After leaving the office and feeling confident that the X-ray was probably not needed, I reflected on the interaction and while appreciating his honesty with me, I wondered: how many thousands of times per day does something like this happen in any doctor's office and the patient just does what the doctor says and gets unnecessary treatments because it is "protocol"?

We like to describe to our practice members the medical "bus ride" that they and their children are on for a lifetime, which drives them to an early grave. At each bus stop, everyone gets out and does what the medical authorities tell them. The first stop is for vaccines in early childhood The next stop is for pills, shots, lotions and potions. If you stay on the bus, the next stop will be for medical procedures, treatments and surgery. The final stop is an early check-in to the nursing home.

Have you recently been to a hospital or nursing home and seen older folks with dementia, Alzheimer's, or chronic health issues? Did you ever stop and ask yourself or think about what you're doing differently with your health so you don't end up like them? They bought a ticket on the medical bus and made all the stops.

Are you on that same medical bus? Are you getting your shots, treatments, pills and surgery too? How can we expect our babies and children to grow up healthy if we keep doing the same things that made us or these other people become so sick and diseased? We recommend you switch bus lines and get on the bus that takes you on the health and healing route, the healthy, inside-out, body designed by God route that we all desire.

We find in our practice that many parents research the benefits of the inside-out approach only after they've had a medical error, drug, or vaccine reaction. In some cases it's a problem of "too little, too late." Thank God they trust us with their baby's health needs and now want "health-care" instead of "sick-care," but parents need to research the type of health care and health choices they will give their newborn baby before a reaction or problem occurs.

There is nothing wrong with researching the car seat or crib they are planning on buying for the baby, but have they spent similar amounts of time researching or studying the type of birth they will be having, or the vaccines they will be injecting into their newborn's bloodstream? Most parents spend countless hours picking out paint colors, cribs and furnishings for the nursery, but take with blind faith what the doctor says about the medical treatment for themselves and their baby.

We wish they made a Consumer Reports on "Hospitals, Doctors and Drugs." If they did, parents would realize the potential damage that could be done and chiropractic offices like ours would be caring for and adjusting 95 percent (or more) of the newborns instead of less than five percent, like we are now. The cliché we always say in chiropractic is, "If parents knew what we know, they would do what we do"—natural health and healing God's way, allowing the innate intelligence that God put inside the body to fully and freely express itself.

As the research continues to reveal the heavy burden that pharmaceutical medical care places upon all of us, including our precious babies and pregnant moms, we pray that you will join this movement. We want to share the knowledge of health and healing God's way, from the inside out and let every mother or expecting mother know that their baby was wonderfully and magnificently designed by God..

> *The doctor of the future will give no medicine, but will interest his patients in the care of the human frame and in the cause and prevention of disease.*
>
> — Thomas Edison

> *The physician of tomorrow will have no interest in pathology or morbid anatomy, for his study will be in health. The prognosis of disease will no longer depend on physical signs and symptoms but on the ability of the patient to harmonize himself with his spiritual life.*
>
> —Dr. Edward Bach — Bacteriologist

Eli's Birth Story
By Trecia Wells

My husband and I had been married for ten years and we had been trying to get pregnant the entire time. The doctor said I was infertile. We went as far as getting insemination but did not do Clomid shots or in vitro, feeling those options were not right for us, as Clomid in particular can force the body to do something it may not be prepared to do. However, we still wanted children, so seven years into our marriage, we adopted a baby from birth. After we adopted, I told God in my prayer time that I was settled and comfortable with how things were and that I was happy and content. But He had a different plan for me.

Despite what the doctors told us, ten years into our marriage and ten years into trying, I began to conceive. The first baby I conceived, I lost six weeks into my pregnancy. Seven months later, I conceived again with my son, Eli. I was 36 when I got pregnant and 37 when I birthed Eli. In medical protocol, I was considered "high risk" because of my age, my infertile past and my previous miscarriage. Although all these facts were true, I never felt that way. I felt healthy. I believed God would finish what He had started.

In all the years that I had dreamed about being pregnant, my experience while carrying Eli was not what I expected. My OB at the time and people around me kept filling me with fear. They poured the "what ifs" into my head and during each doctor's visit I was poked and prodded. Four months into the pregnancy we decided to leave our OB and contact a midwife. Once we left, we never looked back.

I wanted a birth that was not treated as an emergency. I wanted to birth at home with a midwife, where the baby could be free of stress and I could have him by natural means. I was physically fit, ate well and was mentally prepared; I knew I could do this. I walked three miles every day while I was pregnant and on the day of the due date, I had walked a mile and a half. My birth with Eli was amazing. I delivered him with my midwife at her birthing center. I was in labor for 12 hours: I left my house that morning at 10:20 am and returned home at 10:23 pm with my baby in hand. It was a wonderful first pregnancy.

My next pregnancy was a completely different experience. When I first got pregnant, my midwife was concerned about the measurements taken of my belly. Either we were incorrect about the date of conception, or we had another situation on our hands. I kept measuring bigger and bigger without a lot of movement from within my belly. I went to get a sonogram to confirm what our situation was. We came to find out I was pregnant with twins.

My midwife could not legally deliver twins, so we were forced to explore different options. We did our research and found an OB who was skilled in doing natural births for twins. Unfortunately, he was a great distance from our home. He also insisted that I visit weekly to monitor the babies and for monograms, which my husband and I viewed as unnecessary and excessive. We understood the usefulness of these practices, but saw them only needed in emergency situations. We did not want to expose our babies to instruments that could potentially harm them. We asked the OB if we could sign a waiver to bypass the practices, but he told us that he could not care for us if we did.

From this point, my husband and I prayed, researched and decided we would birth from home, just the two of us. We felt our babies deserved a peaceful entry into this world. We knew complications could arise, especially with twins, but we found peace and reassurance from God. In my prayer time with Him, He revealed five things about the birthing of my twins. He told me to have peace and that there was a plan in place for their birth. My babies would be born head down, they would weigh around 7 pounds, I would birth them vaginally, they would be boys and God told me the day when they would be born.

More reading and research began. I read book after book. I monitored my urine, ordered test strips online, made sure my sugars and proteins were right, exercised and ate nutritionally. As the pregnancy went by, people were concerned with our choice to deliver at home and began to tell horror stories. These stories began to wear on me emotionally and mentally. I knew I was not the first woman to ever have her baby at home and I wouldn't be the last. I stayed strong by focusing on the positive stories: the stories of women who had birthed triplets at home and by natural means.

At 37 weeks one of my babies was head up. But God had told me they would be head down. I began to doubt myself and question if what we were doing was right. At 38 weeks, however, that baby flipped. I thought there was no room in there for this to happen, but when it did I woke up from my sleep and thought I was in labor. I knew he had flipped that morning based on where I read his heart beat. My stethoscope revealed that it was below my belly button, which meant he was head down.

From this point things began to fall in line with what God had told me. Week 39 came and I put myself on bed rest because the twins had gotten so heavy that I was unable to control my bladder. On week 40, I began to feel contractions. They hit at 3 am on Friday morning. At times they were regular, while other times they were sporadic. The contractions lasted the entire day until 3 am on Saturday. They lasted for 24 hours and then all of a sudden they stopped. They started back up again that day and lasted until the following day, but still were not regular. Finally, on Sunday night, my water broke and within 20 minutes I had my first solid contraction. Because it was so early in the morning, my other two boys had been sleeping and they awoke to the sounds of me pushing. They came into the room in time for my delivery. My first twin, Titus, came out at 4:10 am weighing 7 pounds 3 ounces and as soon as he came out, I knew my next twin coming out would be a boy. Levi was born 13 minutes after Titus. Everything God had told my heart came true; the weight, the day, the gender of my babies and the means by which they were born.

So there we were with four boys. Family and friends began to ask if we planned to have another. "No, no, no," I thought. But God began to tug on my heart. When we visited family friends for Thanksgiving, we were chatting with one another when the question came up: "What would you say is the answer to all life's problems?" Our friends responded, "Have more babies!"

We knew then that it was in our future to get pregnant again. With that, I was pregnant within the first month of trying. I contacted our midwife and we started our appointments. I was surprised to find out that I was pregnant with twins again.

During the sonogram appointment, they told me one baby was healthy and strong, while the other didn't look like it was going to make it. The unhealthy baby would undergo vanishing twin syndrome, where the tissues would be absorbed and used as nutrients. When I heard this news, I thought, "What do I do with that?" I mourned for about a month for the baby I would never hold and then turned to celebrate the baby that God had given us.

When I had Lilly, it was another beautiful birthing experience. I had no complications, even though I was into my 40s. The day Lilly came, I started having contractions in the morning that lasted until she was birthed. I went to my midwife's clinic with contractions one minute apart, but I was sent home because I was only dilated one centimeter. The day continued, as well as the contractions. I visited the grocery store, the mall and walked around the neighborhood before I went back to the clinic. Finally the time came and I was ready. I wanted to have Lilly in the water, so my midwife filled up the tub. Then, at 12:26 am, during the pushes of all pushes, she was out. Lilly came flying out into the water and I scooped her up and held her to my chest.

My husband and I are now happy parents of five wonderful children. I went from being a woman who was told she could never get pregnant to one that birthed four beautiful children.

During all of my pregnancy experiences, I felt that they had rough beginnings, but amazing endings. With Eli I bled in the beginning, which struck me with fear that I would lose him. With my twins there were the legal complications with my midwife and where I would birth them and with Lilly I had to accept the loss of her twin and rejoice in the life God did give me. My pregnancies have been faith-building walks. I had to believe in my body and the way God created it. I was comforted by God during my prayer time and trusted that He would finish what He had begun.

When bringing my babies into this world, we wanted it to be a peaceful experience and not treated as an emergency. Although this culture does not support the way that we chose, we knew it was right for us. Many women don't understand that they have a choice in the way that they birth their baby. They believe that an epidural and other medical procedures are the only way. But women *do* have a choice and their bodies are capable of natural birth. These are the truths that I held onto during the miraculous births of my four babies.

12.

Giving Hope of a Better Way

History has a way of repeating itself. Countless cases in birthing and rearing children point to repeated mistakes and mishaps in this generation it seems unbelievable! The idea that "man (or doctor) knows best," that men prevail over our God-given, natural instincts, just never resonated with either of us. So many abandon the innate wisdom God gave women in birthing and in parents raising their children drug-free, chemical-free and nerve interference free. We can't just stand by and do nothing about this.

Teaching people that there is a better way, giving hope to parents and doing our part to help people make sense of pregnancy, birthing and raising kids naturally is our cause and why we are so passionate about the "Designed by God" series. We believe there is a better way. We believe God bestowed on each of us to do things the right way, His way. We also believe that making sense of the complicated and challenging situations surrounding birthing and raising children naturally is a gift God gave us and reason enough to help people be confident, clear and inspired in their decision making regarding the health of their precious children.

We see things clearly with our family, with the way we raise our children naturally and drug-free. We desire every parent to have clarity and to be confident in whichever direction they choose for their children. We believe the natural God given methods make much more sense; they may go against the grain of society, but that's okay with us, as long as we know it's the right thing to do for ourselves and our children.

The good news is that more and more families are realizing that processed, microwaved, drugged and toxic choices for their family are not the right way, especially long-term. Now more than ever, women are seeking out natural birth options and parents are researching the use and methodology of standard vaccination in America. More families are turning to natural, specific chiropractic care as their primary source of care for the family. More people are choosing organic and natural foods. More people are picking up books like this one and getting educated, discovering why they are doing the things they do and taking responsibility for their health and the health of their loved ones.

We sometimes call ourselves hope dealers and not dope dealers! We wanted to share a list of the most important things we personally do and recommend to provide more hope for you and your family now and in the future.

1. Get yourself and your family checked for nerve interference by a principled specific chiropractor, as spinal nerve interference is detrimental to human health.
2. Protect your family's health by buying Organic and non-GMO groceries, at least as much as possible to rid your

food of pesticides, hormones, antibiotics and a multitude of other chemicals.

3. Switch your home cleaning chemicals and your cosmetics to toxin-free brands so you can have a chemical-free home and body.

4. Research and get educated about vaccinations and other harmful drugs, whether over-the-counter or prescribed and learn of the harmful side effects and adverse reactions they cause.

5. If you're expecting or planning a baby, get informed on all types of birthing practices and start thinking about what your birth plan would look like.

6. Make it a habit to STOP eating processed and fast foods. You would never give your child a cigarette! See fast food in the same way.

7. Unplug your microwave. Dare to prepare fresh food!

8. Read labels, not just fat or calories, but look for artificial sweeteners, MSG, high fructose corn syrup, artificial colors and other additives that just aren't good for you and damage your body. Avoid them like the plague.

9. Stop listening to well-meaning friends, family, doctors and the media about what they think or say "health care" is, because the vast majority of them are living a drugged, toxic and unhealthy outside-in lifestyle.

10. Utilize the *Baby Designed by God* resource guide, encourage others to read the book and get informed, plugged in and take action steps today to start living from the inside out.

These are some of the things that we do on a daily basis that have helped our family be healthy, happier and drug free. About eight years ago, we really committed to being better with our health, our choices in food and the things we put in and on our bodies.

We'd love to tell you there is an overnight fix, but when making the best decisions for you and your family, sometimes you end up on the road less traveled. It may seem like a detour that initially takes longer, but the time and financial investment reaps health dividends in the years to come.

Remember that there is a better way, filled with hope of a healthier tomorrow for you and your family. We believe in you and are looking forward to hearing your testimonies and success stories. Please send us an email or share them with us on Facebook!

stories@designed-by-god.com
www.facebook.com/DesignedByGodBook

Living from the Inside-Out,
Drs. Amanda & Jeremy Hess

Baby Designed by God
Resource Guide

BIRTHING OPTIONS:

Lamazeinternational.org—A great source to get informed on birthing. You can watch webinars and videos, learn healthy birth practices, network with other moms and more. The Lamaze Healthy Birth Practices help simplify the birth process with a natural approach that helps alleviate fears and manage pain. Regardless of the baby's size, labor's length and complexity, or the mother's confidence level, these care practices will help keep labor and birth as safe and healthy as possible.

Cfmidwifery.org—Looking for a midwife? Or just trying to find out the role of a midwife in the birthing process? You've come to the right place! Citizens for Midwifery is the only national consumer-based group that promotes the *midwives model of care*. CfM provides information and resources that promote the local *midwife*, as well as *midwives* and *midwifery* care across the country.

Bradleybirth.com—This is a great birthing method and I love the Bradley Method's mission and vision of their classes, which stress the importance of healthy baby, healthy mother and healthy families. Their goal is to attract families who are willing to take the responsibility needed for preparation and birth. They think that natural childbirth is an important goal since most people want to give their babies every possible advantage, without the side effects of drugs given during labor and birth. Bradley Method® classes teach families how to have natural births.

Birthcenters.org—The American Association of Birth Centers promotes and supports birth centers as a means to uphold the rights of healthy women and their families, in all communities, to birth their children in an environment that is safe, sensitive and cost-effective, with minimal intervention.

Mymidwife.org—The American College of Nurse-Midwives has embarked on an ambitious plan to help the United States refocus on and improve women's health care services and, as a result, women's health. Their website is a great resource to find a midwife and it aims to redefine how women understand the health care options available to them. It reveals truths about the value of midwifery care and dispels myths about midwives in the United States and it also describes the education and experience that midwives bring as providers of women's health care.

ICEA.org—A great site to find a doula, childbirth educator, or a birthing class, the International Childbirth Education Association (ICEA) is a professional organization that supports educators and health care professionals who believe in freedom to make decisions based on knowledge of alternatives in family-centered maternity and newborn care.

Dona.org—Dona is a good place to find a doula, or simply to discover what a doula does and if you might need one for your birth. Their organization supports doulas who strive to help women and their partners to have satisfying childbirth and postpartum experiences.

Earthmotherbirth.com—Holistic birth consultants who help you get excited about giving birth naturally.

Waterbirthinfo.com—This waterbirth website provides in-depth information on the use of water for labor, childbirth and early childhood development. If you've thought you might want a waterbirth, exploring this site is a must!

Happyhealthychild.com—This 4-DVD set brings the wisdom, expertise and insights of more than 30 world-renowned experts from all fields of science and health on topics about pregnancy, birthing and having a happy, healthy child.

BREAST FEEDING:

Lalecheleague.org—The mission of La Leche League International is to help mothers worldwide to breastfeed through mother-to-mother support, encouragement, information and education, as well as to promote a better understanding of breastfeeding as an important element in the healthy development of the baby and mother. Their website is a fantastic resource for mothers and anyone wanting to learn about the essentials of breastfeeding or to get help with breastfeeding.

Breastfeedingonline.com—This is a really good place to find answers to all those questions while breastfeeding. The website hopes to help empower women to make the choice to breastfeed and to educate society at large about the importance and benefits of breastfeeding.

Kellymom.com—This is a mother-driven website about simple questions we all might have about breastfeeding, as well as many blogs about different topics. Their goal is to provide support and evidence-based information on breastfeeding, sleep and parenting.

Breastfeedingbasics.com—This website handles some of the tough issues surrounding breastfeeding and is the right place to find answers to your breastfeeding questions and practical solutions to any breastfeeding problems you may encounter as you nurse your baby.

GOAT'S MILK & ALTERNATIVES:

Mtcapra.com—The "Goat Milk Experts," Mt. Capra specializes in producing high quality goat milk products. They produce goat milk protein supplements, as well as mineral and sports drink supplements. Many of their products and powders are suitable for making infant formula. Check out their website to see how goat milk and human milk are very close in chemical structure.

Meyenberg.com—A company with a great vision, it provides excellent goat products for you and your baby and it is a great source for infant formula that provides good nutrition, which is a much better choice than dairy- or soy-based formulas.

Nationalmilkbank.org & Hmbana.org—Both are milk banks and places to connect if you either want to donate milk, or are in need of milk for particular reasons.

NATURAL HEALTH TOPICS:

Mercola.com—The world's #1 natural health website. Dr. Mercola's mission is to educate and provide simple, inexpensive tools to help limit or avoid expensive and potentially dangerous drugs and surgery. Make sure you sign up for Dr. Mercola's free email newsletters that will keep you up-to-date on healthy living.

Naturalnews.com—We highly recommend Mike Adams' email newsletter and his website for articles and research about health, longevity, foods and natural remedies. He even addresses those "fringe" topics no one else likes to talk about publicly, such as what's really in the foods you're buying and how corporate American food suppliers are deceiving us on a daily basis.

Ewg.org—The Environmental Working Group is the nation's leading environmental health research and advocacy organization. Their mission is to serve as a watchdog to see that Americans get straight facts, unfiltered and unspun, so they can make healthier choices and enjoy a cleaner environment. As we talk about in the book, their SKIN DEEP Cosmetic Safety Database (ewg.org/skindeep) is a must for every mother who really wants to know what's in the products she is putting in and on her children and the family!

Flouridealert.org—This website will transform how you think about and use fluoride. The website itself is very user-friendly and interactive, plus it's sure to "upset" your current belief system on fluoride use for yourself and your children.

Holisticmoms.org—The Holistic Moms Network™ is a non-profit organization connecting parents who are interested in holistic health and green living. They encourage moms to trust their instincts, parent from the heart, use their innate sense of what is best for their children, live in balance with the Earth and learn about the pros and cons of all health care and parenting options.

Pathwaystofamilywellness.org—Pathways to Family Wellness envisions a world of thriving, empowered families who easily connect to inner and outer resources, practitioners and a supportive community needed to create wholeness on all levels of existence. This site offers extensive articles, research and data on healthy living for the whole family. Their magazine is a must to subscribe to—it's one of our favorites and we give them out to out practice members.

Responsibletechnology.org—This is another great website for the above average consumer who wants to know the truth on food resources, fraud, corporate and government cover-ups and topics like autism, GMOs and more.

Citizens.org—Citizens for Health (CFH), the "Consumer Voice of the Natural Health Community," is one of the nation's most respected and powerful, consumer action groups dedicated to providing a voice and a platform for informed and effective health activism. Founded in 1992, CFH is a non-profit organization that provides credible and well-researched consumer news, action alerts and opportunities to protect and expand access to innovative dietary supplements, healthy food, non-toxic products and integrative healthcare.

CHIROPRACTIC & NATURAL HEALTH PROVIDERS:

Icpa4kids.com—The International Chiropractic Pediatric Association supports lifetime chiropractic care for the whole family and the site includes research, articles and an easy "doctor finder" to help you find a chiropractor in your area. ICPA is an organization of chiropractic family practitioners dedicated to advancing public awareness and attainment of the chiropractic family lifestyle.

Chiropractic.org—The International Chiropractors Association is a good resource to find a chiropractor anywhere in the world. It represents Doctors of Chiropractic from around the world and maintains and promotes chiropractic's unique identity as a non-therapeutic, drugless and surgical-free health science, based on its fundamental principles and philosophy.

Ifcochiro.org—The mission of the International Federation of Chiropractors and Organizations is to protect, promote and advance chiropractic as a separate and distinct profession dedicated to the detection and correction of vertebral subluxation and spinal nerve interference for the better expression of life.

Hpakids.org—The Holistic Pediatric Alliance is an educational organization. They aim to unite parents and health professionals in the common goal of improving and transforming family health care into a safe, nurturing and sensible holistic system. They empower parents to trust their natural wisdom and make informed choices on behalf of their children.

Naturopathic.org—Naturopathic physicians combine the wisdom of nature with the rigors of modern science. Steeped in traditional healing methods, principles and practices, naturopathic medicine focuses on holistic, proactive prevention and comprehensive diagnosis and treatment. By using protocols that minimize the risk of harm, naturopathic physicians help facilitate the body's inherent ability to restore and maintain optimal health. It is the naturopathic physician's role to identify and remove barriers to good health by helping to create a healing internal and external environment.

Homeopathic.org—Homeopathy is a form of natural health methods that work to heal the body, rather than simply treat an illness's symptoms. It is extremely safe to use (even with very small children), very affordable, made from natural products and FDA-approved and it has none of the side effects of many traditional medications.

FOODS:

Foodmatters.tv—*Food Matters* features a plethora of information on natural health topics, nutrition-rich recipes and interviews with leading health experts who reveal the best natural healing choices you can make for you and your family's health.

Foodidentitytheft.com—Food Identity Theft alerts consumers about threats to the food we buy for ourselves and our families. The Food Identity Theft Project for Citizens for Health believes Americans have the right to know what ingredients are in the food products they consume. Food Identity Theft provides important facts to consumers about food safety issues, as well as ways to connect with Congress and government regulators to express their opinions and concerns about truthful food policies.

Superhealthykids.com—The goal of Super Healthy Kids is to educate families to become healthier. With the proper knowledge, experience, tools and resources, we can begin making changes to create a healthier generation of kids. Super Healthy Kids offers all kinds of recipes, baby food ideas, meal plans and dishes for kids and advice and ideas for everything from picky eaters to eating for a healthy pregnancy.

Westonaprice.org—This foundation is dedicated to restoring nutrient-dense foods to the human diet through education, research and activism. It supports a number of movements that contribute to this objective, including accurate nutrition instruction, organic and biodynamic farming, pasture-feeding of livestock, community-supported farms, honest and informative labeling, prepared parenting and nurturing therapies. Check out some of their nutrition and food lists and recommendations.

Organicconsumers.org—This is a very informative website if you want to explore and know what's beneath the surface on organic foods, food safety, children's health, genetic engineering, corporate accountability and more.

Fooddemocracynow.org—This grassroots movement of more than 650,000 farmers and citizens is dedicated to building a sustainable food system that protects our natural environment, sustains farmers and nourishes families. They really tell it like it is—there's no political correctness on this website!

Cornucopia.org—This is an interesting website explaining where our food comes from and it seeks to protect sustainable and local farming and organic agriculture.

HERBS, HOMEOPATHIC & NATURAL REMEDIES:

Herballegacy.com—This is a fantastic site for quickly looking up herbal remedies for your baby or family. Learn the "secrets" of natural healing directly from the writings and teachings of Dr. John R. Christopher, America's pioneer in herbal medicine.

Learningherbs.com—The Gallagher family shares their wealth of knowledge on herbs and natural remedies. Much of what they recommend on their site are remedies and recipes they use themselves. They believe it is so important in this day and age for families to be in control of their day-to-day health care. They want to spread knowledge that will help people stay healthy and empower them with skills to treat common illnesses naturally.

Earthclinic.com—This is an informative website that has multiple natural health writers and contributors posting on health and hope through safe, inexpensive, natural cures and home remedies to people around the world.

VACCINES:

NVIC.org—Barbara Loe Fisher, the founder of the National Vaccine Information Center, has been at the front line fighting for children and families of vaccine-injured children long before this subject became well known. NVIC launched the vaccine safety and informed consent movement in America in the early 1980s and is the oldest and largest consumer-led organization advocating for the institution of vaccine safety and informed consent protections in the public health system.

Thinktwice.com—The Thinktwice Global Vaccine Institute was established in 1996 to provide parents and other concerned people with educational resources enabling them to make more informed vaccine decisions. Thinktwice encourages an uncensored exchange of vaccine information, supports every family's right to accept or reject vaccines and offers many good, short books on explaining all the ins and outs of vaccination.

Vactruth.com—The father of a vaccine-injured child created this website. It provides a great source of information when making decisions on this vitally important topic. Sign up and get the "vaccine ingredient summary" that they provide for free.

RECOMMENDED MOVIES & DOCUMENTARIES:

The Business of Being Born
www.thebusinessofbeingborn.com
A must watch for every natural minded person as it will reveal not only why you would want to have as natural of a birth as possible, but also the unfortunate reality of pregnancy and birthing being run like a business in a hospital setting.

Born in the USA
www.patchworksfilms.net/films/born_usa.html
This film gives an up close and in-depth view of all sides of birthing and answers many questions and myths the average consumer has about pregnancy.

It's My Body, My Baby, My Birth
www.itsmybodymybabymybirth.com
This is a great documentary that will walk you through multiple couples' birthing experiences and their individual situations and stories.

Natural Born Babies
www.naturalbornbabies.com
Natural Born Babies presents a modern account of today's natural childbirth. Told by ten mothers, this short film chronicles their journeys to challenge the conventional hospital birth model to give birth in their own way.

The Greater Good
www.greatergoodmovie.org
This is a very well-produced documentary on vaccines, the industry behind them and specific topics like autism, vaccine reactions and Gardisil awareness.

Doctored: The Film the AMA Does Not Want You to See
www.doctoredthemovie.com
This is an intriguing documentary about the inner workings of the medical profession and how chiropractic and other natural health providers and services can provide solutions to so many people who have lost all hope.

Food, Inc.
www.takepart.com/foodinc/film
Hungry for change? If you watch this movie, you will never view your dinner the same way again! In *Food, Inc.*, filmmaker Robert Kenner lifts the veil on our nation's food industry, exposing the highly mechanized underbelly that has been hidden from the American consumer with the consent of our government's regulatory agencies, the USDA and FDA.

Food Matters – "Food is better medicine than drugs"
www.foodmatters.tv
This is another excellent documentary on food and our food supply, with leading experts giving facts and teaching on how our situation is getting worse every day and what you need to know and can do about it for you and your family.

Got the facts on Milk? *The Milk Documentary*
www.milkdocumentary.com
This is a must for all moms to watch, as most of us believe that milk is good for us, or at least that's what the dairy industry has been telling us all these years. Watch the truth for yourself and protect your family!

Super Size Me
This was one of the first "food" documentaries to examine our food supply and how questionable it is becoming. The documentary chronicles a man who eats only McDonald's food for 30 days and tracks the drastic effect it has on his physical and psychological well-being. It also explores the fast food industry's corporate influence, including how it encourages poor nutrition for its own profit.

BOOKS WORTH READING:

NATURAL HEALTH TOPICS:

How to Raise a Healthy Child in Spite of Your Doctor
by Robert S. Mendelsohn, M.D.

Prescription for Nutritional Healing, Fifth Edition: A Practical A-to-Z Reference to Drug-Free Remedies Using Vitamins, Minerals, Herbs & Food Supplements
by Phyllis A. Balch CNC

Chiropractic First
by Terry A. Rondberg, D.C.

Vaccines: Are They Really Safe and Effective
by Neil Z. Miller

The Vaccine Guide: Risks and Benefits for Children and Adults
by Randall Neustaedter O.M.D.

Food to Live By: The Earthbound Farm Organic Cookbook
by Myra Goodman, Linda Holland , Pamela McKinstry

The Organic Family Cookbook
by Anni Daulter

Prescription for Natural Cures: A Self-Care Guide for Treating Health Problems with Natural Remedies Including Diet, Nutrition, Supplements and Other Holistic Methods
by James F. Balch and Mark Stengler

The Country Almanac of Home Remedies: Time-Tested & Almost Forgotten Wisdom for Treating Hundreds of Common Ailments, Aches & Pains Quickly and Naturally
by Brigitte Mars and Chrystle Fiedler

BIRTHING BOOKS:

Ina May's Guide to Childbirth
by Ina May Gaskin

Natural Childbirth the Bradley Way: Revised Edition
by Susan McCutcheon and Robert A. Bradley

Spiritual Midwifery
by Ina May Gaskin

The Thinking Woman's Guide to a Better Birth
by Henci Goer

Birthing a Better Way: 12 Secrets for Natural Childbirth
by Kalena Cook and Margaret Christensen, M.D.

The Essential Homebirth Guide: For Families Planning or Considering Birthing at Home
by Jane E. Drichta, Jodilyn Owen and Dr. Christiane Northrup

The Birth Book: Everything You Need to Know to Have a Safe and Satisfying Birth
by William Sears and Martha Sears

BABY FOOD BOOKS:

Babies Bellies: An Organic and Natural Approach to Nourishing Healthy Children: A Homemade Baby Food Cookbook (Volume 1)
by Dawn Marie Klemp

Top 100 Baby Purees
by Annabel Karmel

The Wholesome Baby Food Guide: Over 150 Easy, Delicious and Healthy Recipes from Purees to Solids
by Maggie Meade

201 Organic Baby Purees: The Freshest, Most Wholesome Food Your Baby Can Eat!
by Tamika L. Gardner

The Everything Organic Cooking for Baby and Toddler Book: 300 naturally delicious recipes to get your child off to a healthy start by Kim Lutz and Megan Hart

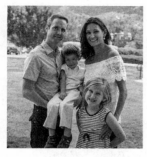

Dr. Jeremy Hess is a practicing chiropractor in Georgia since 2000. He is a graduate of Life University, a member of the Georgia Council of Chiropractic since 1998, a board member since 2007, and serving as Vice President from 2010-2013. He is a member of the International Chiropractic Pediatric Association, National Vaccine Information Center, International Federation of Chiropractors & Organizations and a Lifetime Member of the International Chiropractors Association.

Dr. Amanda Hess is a practicing chiropractor in the state of Georgia since 2003. She completed college as a graduate of the University of South Carolina with a Bachelor's of Science degree in Biology and her Doctorate of Chiropractic degree at Life University. She is a member of the Georgia Council of Chiropractic, League of Chiropractic Women, International Chiropractic Pediatric Association, National Vaccine Information Center, International Federation of Chiropractors & Organizations and a lifetime member of the International Chiropractors Association.

Drs. Jeremy and Amanda Hess own and operate the busiest chiropractic practice in Stockbridge Ga., the busiest in the state and one of the busiest in the world. They also mentor and teach chiropractors and students practice procedures and inspire them to make a huge impact in their communities thru their "AMPED" Mentorship and Development program for chiropractors and natural health providers.

They live in Lake Spivey, GA with their two children, Alyssa and Gabriel. Their mission is to serve God by serving the families of his community and region through principled chiropractic care allowing the Innate healing potential of the body to fully express itself.